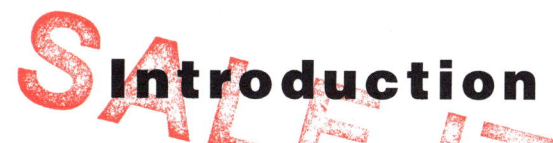

Introduction

Snacktime is a natural time for extending learning, and the recipes in *Teaching Snacks* make it easy for you to do just that. Using this book's nine different topic areas, ranging from shapes to colors to cooperation, you will find fun and easy ways to encourage your children's learning during snacktime.

For example, if you are exploring colors with your children, then serving "Red Berry Parfaits" (recipe on page 11) would be a natural way to extend that exploration to the snack table. If numbers are the theme of the day, letting your children make their own "Number Mix" (recipe on page 22) would be ideal.

Each snack recipe also includes ideas for having your children help prepare the snack. Working together to make a snack provides a great opportunity to talk about and practice good hygiene and kitchen safety. For example, you could make up a chart to show how to wash hands, hang it by your sink, and help your children follow the steps on it.

Snacktime is a relaxed time. It's a time for your children to refuel, socialize, and, with recipes from *Teaching Snacks*, a time for them to learn as well.

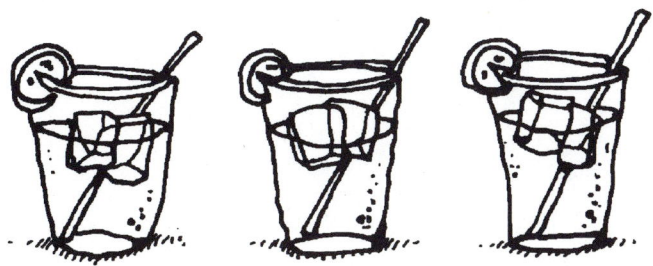

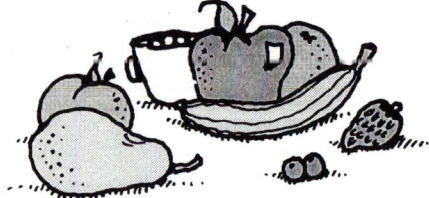

Contents

Cheesy Shapes

¼ cup shredded Monterey Jack cheese
½ cup ricotta cheese
¼ teaspoon garlic powder
¼ teaspoon dried parsley
⅛ teaspoon thyme
Pinch of marjoram
Crackers of various shapes

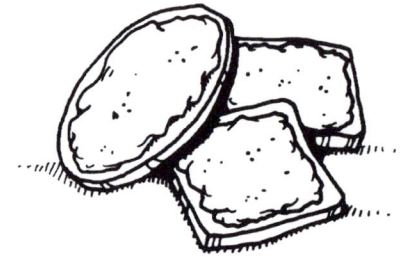

Place shredded cheese and ricotta cheese in a bowl and mix them together with a fork. Add garlic powder, parsley, thyme, and marjoram. Stir until well combined. Spread the cheese mixture on crackers and arrange on a serving tray. Makes ¾ cup of spread.

Cooking Skills

◆ Let your children help shred the Monterey Jack cheese.

◆ Have your children help measure and mix together the cheeses and spices.

◆ Show your children the herbs. Let them smell each one. Ask them to tell you which ones they like best.

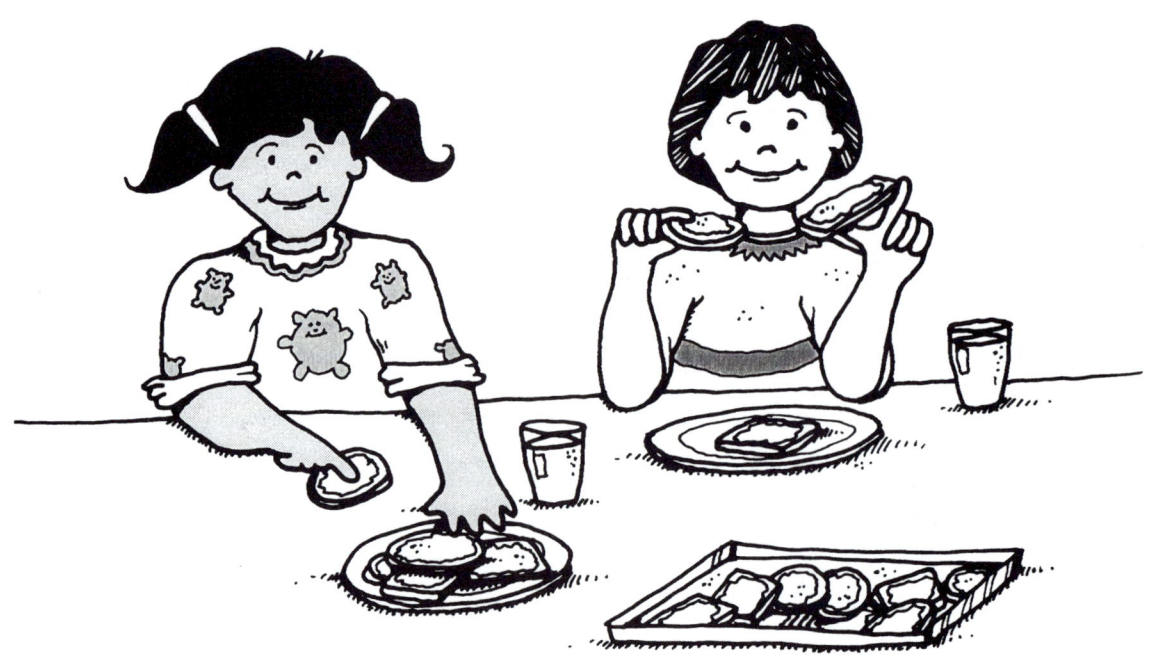

Discovering Shapes

◆ Give each of your children two pairs of shapes. Have him or her find the matching shapes and put them together to make "shape sandwiches."

◆ Let your children select shapes from the tray and name them.

◆ Ask your children to identify the shapes on the serving tray.

◆ Ask your children to select particular shapes from the tray

Finger-Gelatin Shapes

4 cups unsweetened grape juice, divided
4 envelopes unflavored gelatin

Place 1 cup grape juice in a large bowl. Sprinkle gelatin over the juice. Let stand for 1 minute. Heat remaining 3 cups of grape juice to boiling and pour the boiling juice into the gelatin mixture. Stir until gelatin is dissolved. Pour mixture into a greased 9-by-13-inch baking pan. Chill at least 3 hours, until gelatin is firm. Use a sharp knife or cookie cutters to cut the finger gelatin into various shapes. Makes 4 to 5 dozen 2-inch shapes.

Variation: Instead of grape juice, use unsweetened apple juice or other clear juice. (Citrus juices do not work.)

Cooking Skills

◆ Let your children compare the cold and hot juices by feeling the outsides of the measuring cups.

◆ Ask your children to observe the gelatin in its powdered form, after it has absorbed the cold juice, and after the hot juice is added.

◆ Have your children take turns stirring the hot juice mixture to dissolve the gelatin.

◆ Let your children help cut out the shapes or tell you what shapes to cut.

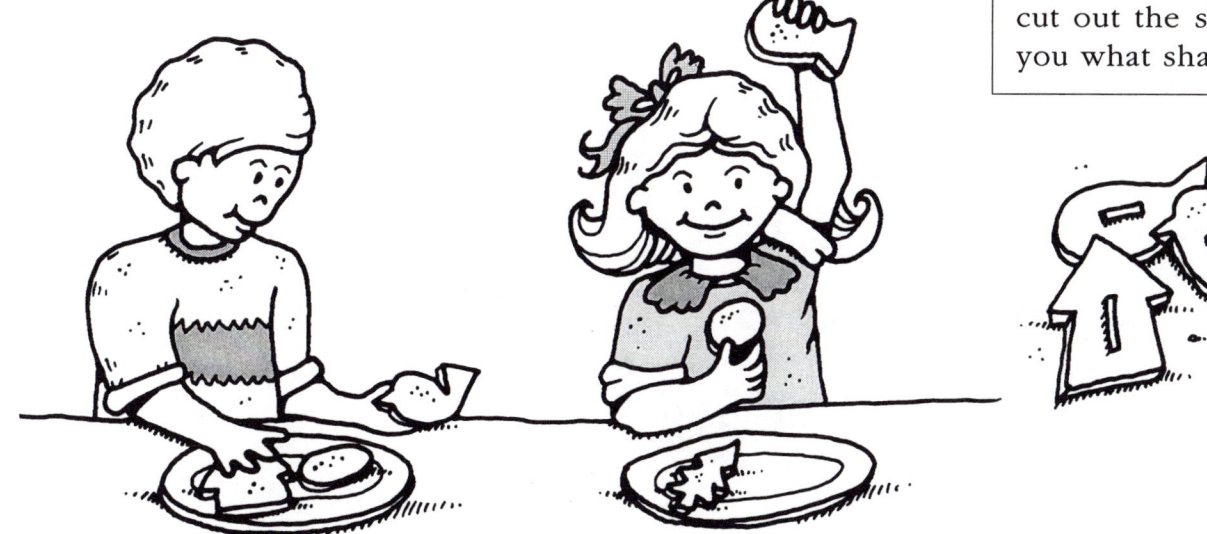

Discovering Shapes

◆ Ask your children to name the shapes you put on their plates.

◆ Let your children select and name the shapes they want.

◆ Give your children several different shapes and let them arrange "shape pictures" on their plates.

◆ Make two batches of gelatin shapes, one with a light-colored juice and one with a dark-colored juice. Give your children several gelatin shapes from each color. Let them sort the shapes on their plates by shape and color before eating them.

Making Shapes

12 ounces Monterey Jack cheese

1 cup stick pretzels

Cut cheese into small cubes. Push the ends of pretzels into cheese cubes to make two-dimensional shapes (squares, triangles, rectangles, etc.). Makes about 12 shapes.

Variation: To make three-dimensional shapes (cubes, pyramids, etc.), use toothpicks instead of pretzels. Be sure to remind your children to remove the toothpicks before eating the cheese.

Note: Monterey Jack cheese works best for this snack because it is softer and less crumbly than other cheeses.

Cooking Skills

◆ Cut the cheese into thick strips. Show your children how to use table knives to cut the strips into cubes.

◆ Have your children put the pretzels in a bowl. Ask them to pick out all the broken ones.

◆ Let one of your children pass out a plate to each child.

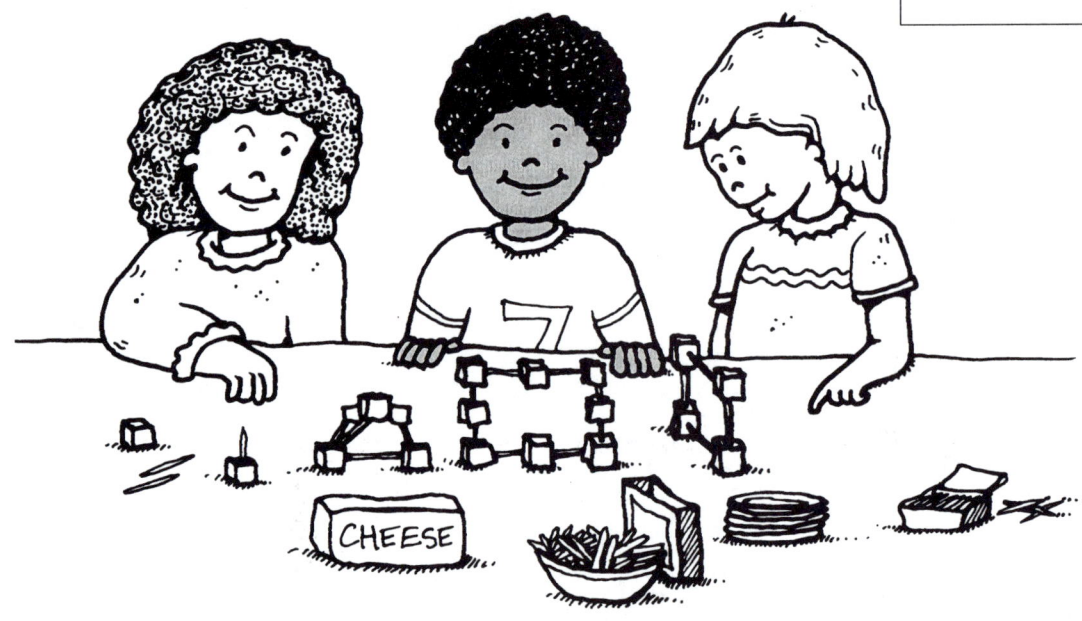

Discovering Shapes

◆ Show your children the cut-up cheese and the pretzels. Ask them if they can name the shape of the cheese (cubes) and the shape of the pretzels (cylinders). Then have them look around the room for other cube and cylinder shapes.

◆ Give each child a plate with six pretzels and six cheese cubes on it. Have the children use the pretzels and cheese cubes to make shapes.

◆ Show your children a square and a triangle (made with pretzels and cheese cubes) and a cube and a pyramid (made with toothpicks and cheese cubes). Have them compare the shapes. Point out the squares in the cubes and the triangles in the pyramids.

◆ Make several shapes with the pretzels and cheese cubes. Ask your children to name each shape.

Puzzling Shapes

Clean a large, thick carrot and a zucchini. Cut the carrot and zucchini crosswise into thin circles. Use a canape cutter (available at kitchen stores) to cut a small shape out of each carrot and zucchini circle. Put the shapes back into the circles to make Puzzling Shapes.

Variation: Instead of a carrot and zucchini, select light- and dark-colored bread slices. Toast the bread and use cookie cutters to cut shapes out of the centers.

Cooking Skills

◆ Let your children observe the carrot and zucchini. Ask them to tell you how they are alike and how they are different.

◆ Have your children clean the vegetables.

◆ Let your children select which canape cutters to use when cutting shapes out of the vegetable circles.

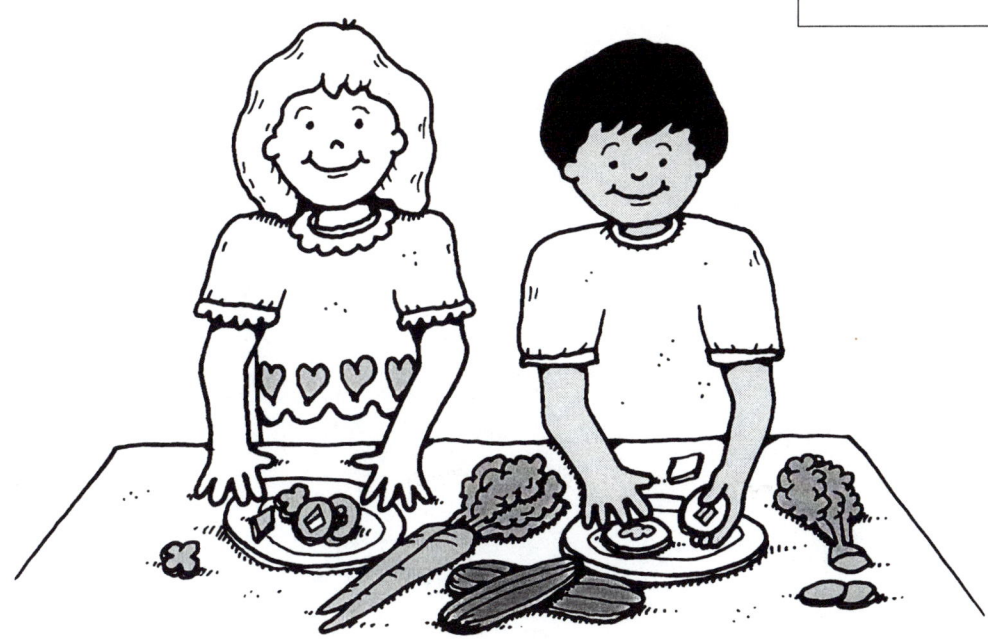

Discovering Shapes

◆ Give each child several Puzzling Shapes. Let them take the shapes in and out of the puzzles.

◆ For each child, arrange a plate with several puzzles that have their shapes set aside. Let your children put the shapes back in the appropriate puzzles.

◆ Give each child a carrot puzzle and a zucchini puzzle with the same shape cut out of them. Let them put the carrot shape in the zucchini puzzle and vice versa.

◆ Ask your children to name the shapes cut out of their puzzles.

Rainbow Salad

1 apple, cored and diced
1 orange, peeled and diced
1 cup grapes, sliced in half
1 banana, sliced
1 cup sliced strawberries
1 cup blueberries
1 cup diced peaches
1 cup diced pears

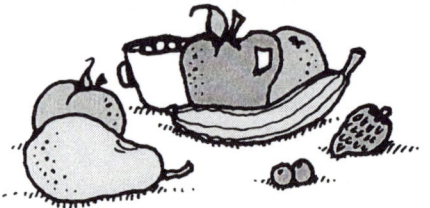

Place fruit pieces in a large bowl. Stir gently to combine. Serve in small bowls or cups. Makes sixteen ½-cup servings.

Cooking Skills

◆ Let your children help wash and peel the fruits.

◆ Give your children table knives and let them help cut the soft fruits.

◆ Put each kind of fruit in a separate bowl. Set out the bowls with individual serving spoons. Give each child a small bowl. Let your children put small amounts of the fruits they want into their bowls to make their own Rainbow Salads.

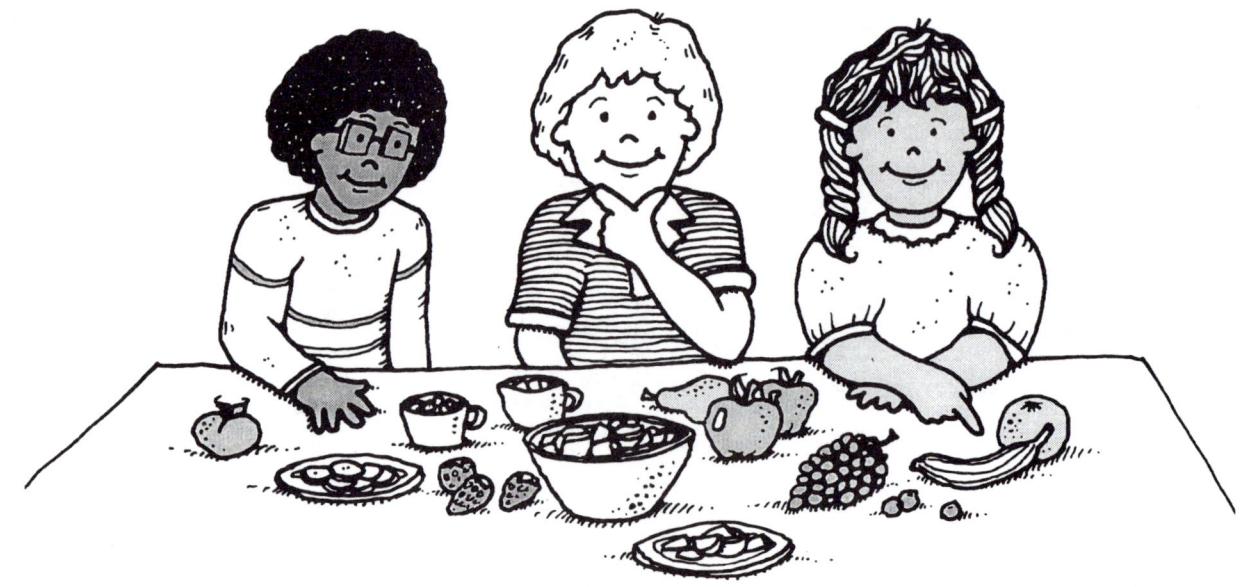

Discovering Colors

◆ Encourage your children to name the colors of the fruits.

◆ Ask your children to point to the red fruits, the green fruits, the orange fruits, and so on.

◆ Have each child tell you his or her favorite color. Ask the child if the same color of fruit is in his or her Rainbow Salad.

Red Berry Parfaits

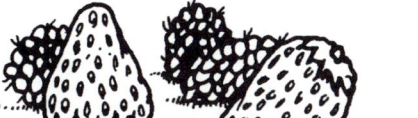

½ cup ricotta cheese
1 ½ tablespoons plain yogurt
1 tablespoon sugar
½ teaspoon vanilla extract
2 cups fresh raspberries or sliced strawberries
Toasted wheat germ or chopped nuts, optional

Place ricotta cheese, yogurt, sugar, and vanilla in a blender container and whirl until smooth. Set out four small clear-plastic cups. In each cup, place 2 tablespoons of berries, add ¼ of the ricotta mixture, then another 2 tablespoons of berries. Garnish with toasted wheat germ or chopped nuts, if desired. Makes 4 parfaits.

Cooking Skills

◆ Have your children help prepare the berries.

◆ Make a recipe chart for the alternating layers of berries and yogurt. Let your children make their own Red Berry Parfaits.

◆ Prepare both kinds of berries. Let your children choose which berries (or combination of berries) they want in their parfaits.

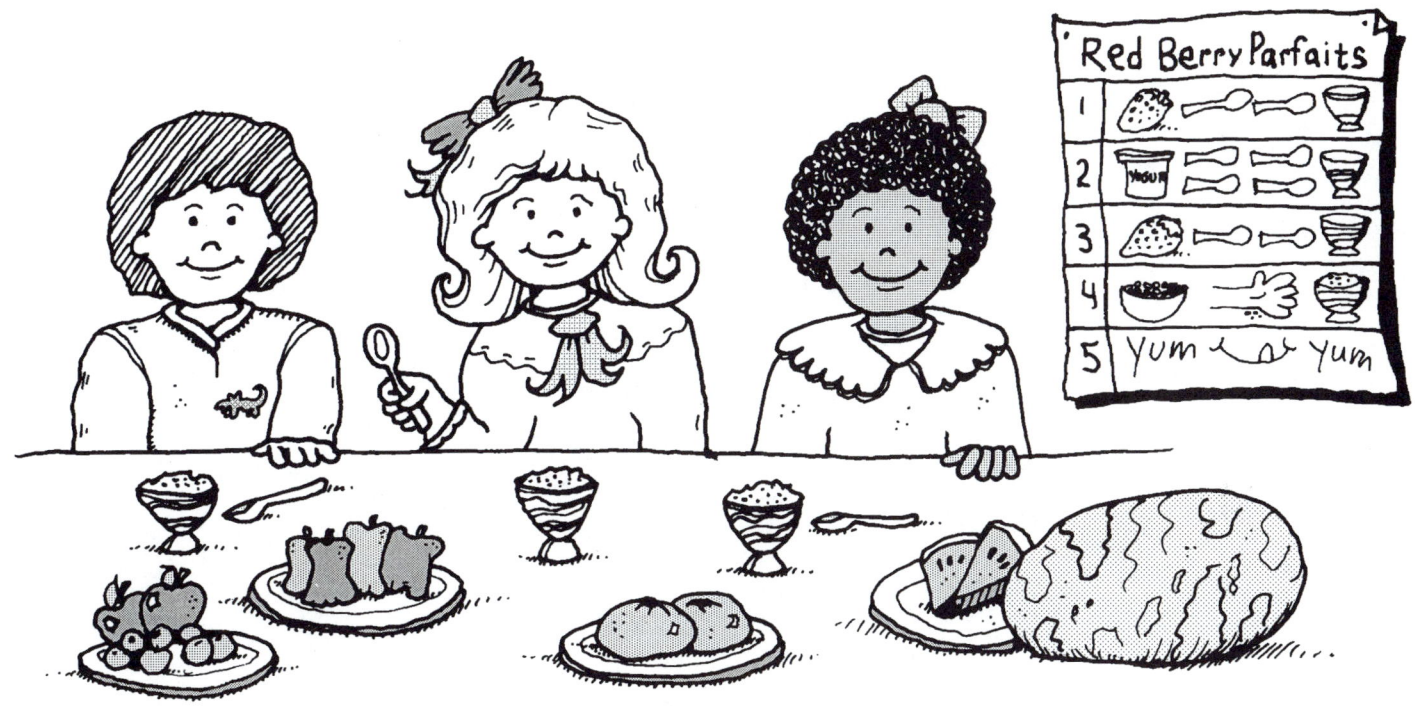

Discovering Colors

◆ Have your children point to the red layers in their parfaits.

◆ Ask your children to name other things around the room that are red.

◆ Set out other red foods such as red apples, watermelon slices, red peppers, tomatoes, and radishes. Let your children name the foods and, if desired, try some of each.

Orange Pops

1 can (6 ounces) unsweetened orange-juice
    concentrate, thawed
¾ cup water
1 cup plain yogurt
1 teaspoon vanilla extract

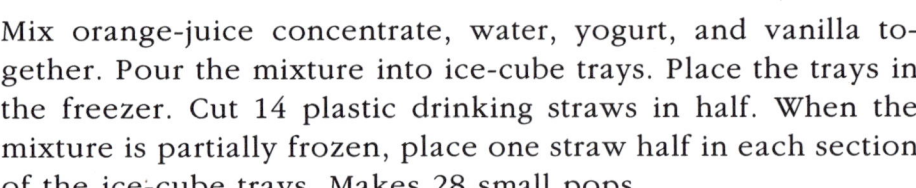

Mix orange-juice concentrate, water, yogurt, and vanilla to-gether. Pour the mixture into ice-cube trays. Place the trays in the freezer. Cut 14 plastic drinking straws in half. When the mixture is partially frozen, place one straw half in each section of the ice-cube trays. Makes 28 small pops.

Cooking Skills

◆ Let your children help measure and mix together the ingredients.

◆ Mark a measuring cup at the ¾-cup level. Fill the empty juice can with wa-ter. Show the children that the water in the can will fill the measuring cup up to the ¾-cup line.

◆ Have your children cut the plastic drinking straws in half.

◆ Let your children place a straw half in each ice-cube section.

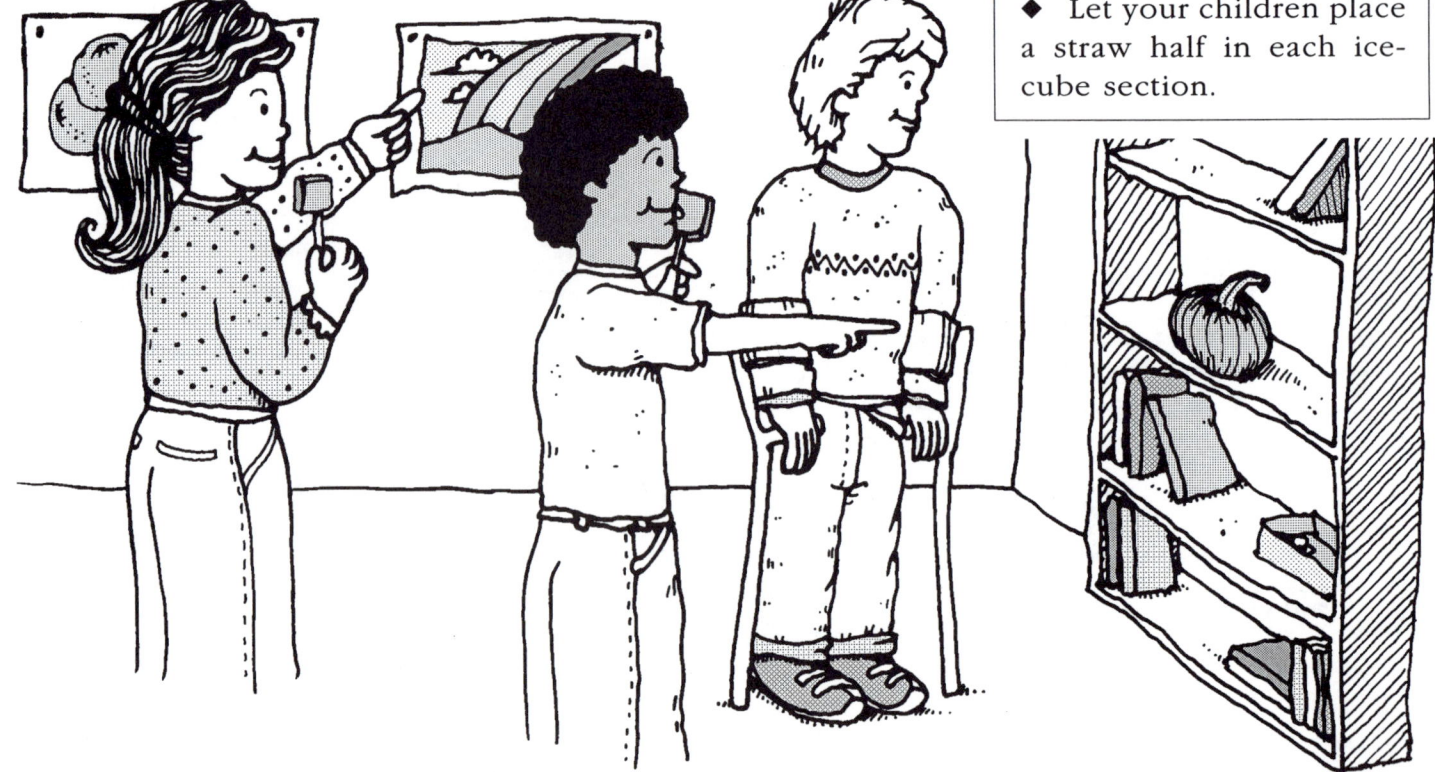

Discovering Colors

◆ Ask your children to tell you the color of the pops.

◆ Have your children point to other things around the room that are orange.

◆ Let your children compare the color of the orange-juice concentrate with the color of the pops. Ask them if they can tell you why the pops are a lighter color.

Yellow Corn Biscuits

1 ¼ cups all-purpose flour
½ cup whole-wheat flour
¾ cup cornmeal
4 teaspoons baking powder
½ teaspoon salt
1 cup buttermilk
¼ cup vegetable oil
1 tablespoon pure maple syrup
¾ cup frozen corn

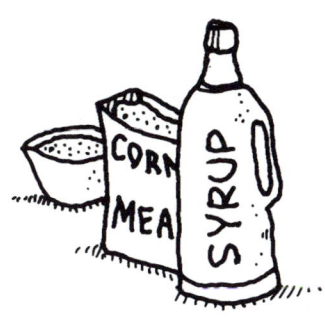

In a large bowl, combine flours, cornmeal, baking powder, and salt. In a separate bowl, mix together buttermilk, oil, and maple syrup. Make a well in the center of the dry ingredients and pour in the buttermilk mixture. Stir just until combined. Gently fold in the corn. Drop by spoonfuls onto a greased baking sheet. Bake at 450°F for 15 minutes or until biscuits are lightly browned. Makes 12 small biscuits.

Cooking Skills

◆ Let your children help measure and mix together the ingredients.

◆ Have your children drop spoonfuls of batter onto the baking sheet.

◆ Purchase some whole dried corn (not popcorn) at a health-food store. Let your children help you grind the corn in a food grinder to make your own cornmeal.

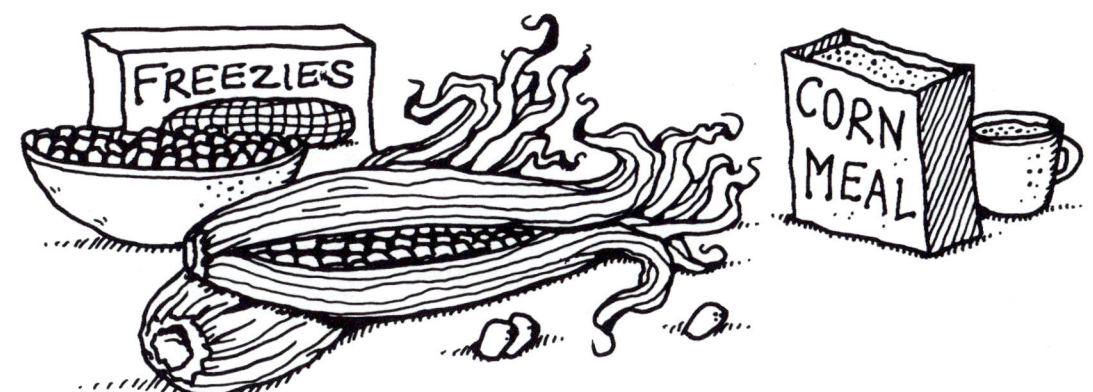

Discovering Colors

◆ Have your children point to the yellow corn in their biscuits.

◆ For a totally yellow treat, let your children eat their yellow biscuits with yellow butter or margarine and golden honey.

◆ Ask your children to name other yellow foods.

◆ Let your children find other objects around the room that are yellow.

◆ Show your children some fresh or frozen corn, dried corn, and cornmeal. Ask them to tell you how the corn items are alike and how they are different.

◆ Let your children look at some ears of Indian corn. Ask them if they can find any yellow kernels on the corn.

Green Salad

Prepare a variety of green vegetables for a salad. Select vegetables such as lettuce, spinach, cabbage, alfalfa sprouts, bell pepper, celery, and broccoli. Mix all the vegetables together in a large bowl to make a Green Salad. Serve the salad with Green Goddess Dressing (recipe follows) on small plates.

Green Goddess Dressing—Mix together ¼ cup mayonnaise, ½ cup yogurt, 1 tablespoon dried parsley, ½ teaspoon chives, ½ teaspoon basil, ⅛ teaspoon salt, dash of garlic powder, and dash of pepper. Makes ¾ cup of dressing.

Cooking Skills

◆ Let your children help wash and prepare the vegetables.

◆ Take your children to the grocery store and let them select green vegetables for your salad.

◆ Let your children help measure and mix together the ingredients for the Green Goddess Dressing. Point out the green herbs.

◆ Have your children take turns using salad forks to toss the green vegetables together in the large bowl.

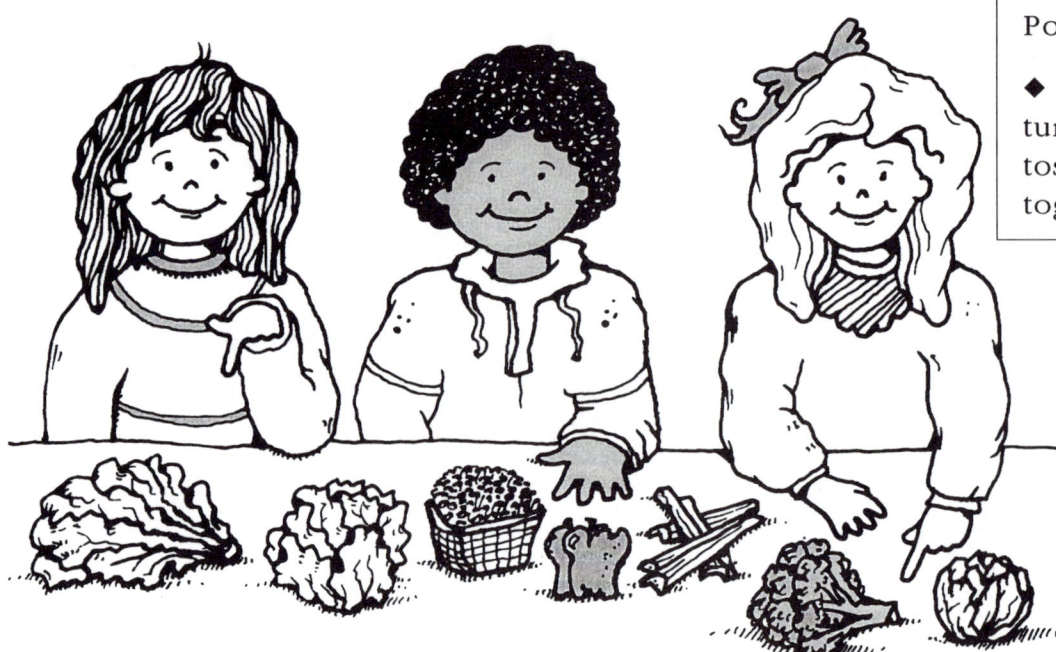

Discovering Colors

◆ Ask your children to notice how many different shades of green are in the Green Salad.

◆ Have your children name other green objects they know.

◆ Show your children whole examples of the cut-up vegetables in the salad. Let them arrange the whole vegetables from darkest to lightest in color.

Blueberry Pancakes

½ cup all-purpose flour
½ cup whole-wheat flour
1 teaspoon baking powder
½ teaspoon baking soda
1 tablespoon vegetable oil
1 egg
1 cup plain yogurt
¼ cup milk
¾ cup blueberries

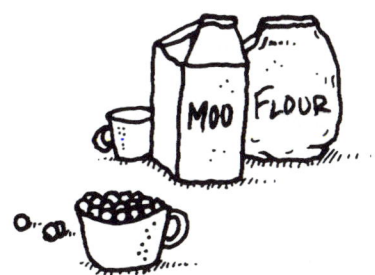

Combine flours, baking powder, and baking soda in a large bowl. In a separate bowl, mix together oil, egg, yogurt, and milk. Add the yogurt mixture to the flour mixture and stir just until combined. Gently fold in blueberries. Spoon small amounts of the batter onto a hot griddle. Makes twelve to fourteen 3-inch pancakes.

Hint: Replace the all-purpose and whole-wheat flours with 1 cup whole-wheat pastry flour (available at health-food stores) for a lighter-tasting pancake.

Cooking Skills

◆ Let your children help measure and mix together the ingredients.

◆ Set out all of the ingredients. Let your children divide the ingredients into two groups, "dry" and "wet."

◆ Let your children watch while you spoon the pancake batter onto the hot griddle. Have them observe what happens to the batter. Ask them to think of reasons why you must use a spatula to turn the pancakes.

◆ Let your children serve the pancakes with a spatula.

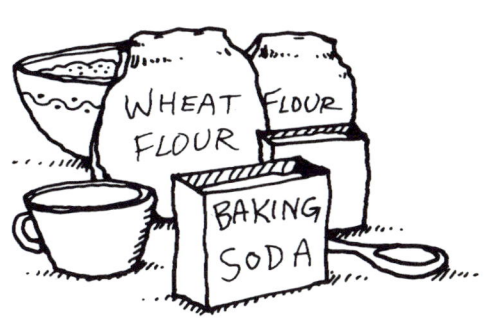

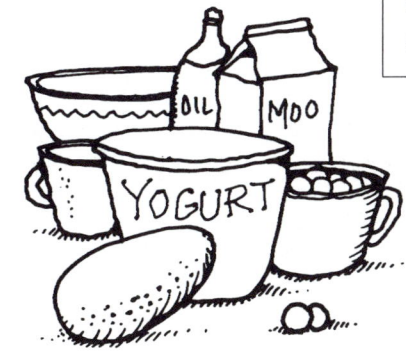

Discovering Colors

◆ Talk with your children about the color blue. Ask them to find the blueberries in their pancakes.

◆ Have your children name other things that are blue.

◆ Let your children count the number of blueberries in their pancakes.

◆ Give each child several uncooked blueberries. Let your children compare the uncooked blueberries with the cooked ones in the pancakes. Ask them to tell you how they are alike and how they are different.

Purple Shake

½ cup plain yogurt
2 teaspoons sugar
½ cup frozen blueberries
½ cup frozen raspberries
¼ teaspoon almond extract

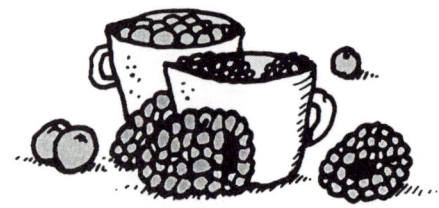

Place yogurt and sugar in a blender container and process until well combined. Add blueberries, raspberries, and almond extract to the yogurt mixture and process until smooth. Makes two ½-cup servings.

Cooking Skills

◆ Have your children watch as you combine the ingredients in the blender. Ask them to predict what will happen to the berries.

◆ Let your children measure out the berries. Ask them to predict which ½ cup will have the largest number of berries. Then have them count the berries in each measuring cup.

◆ Set out small amounts of each of the berries and let your children taste them. Ask them which berries they like the best.

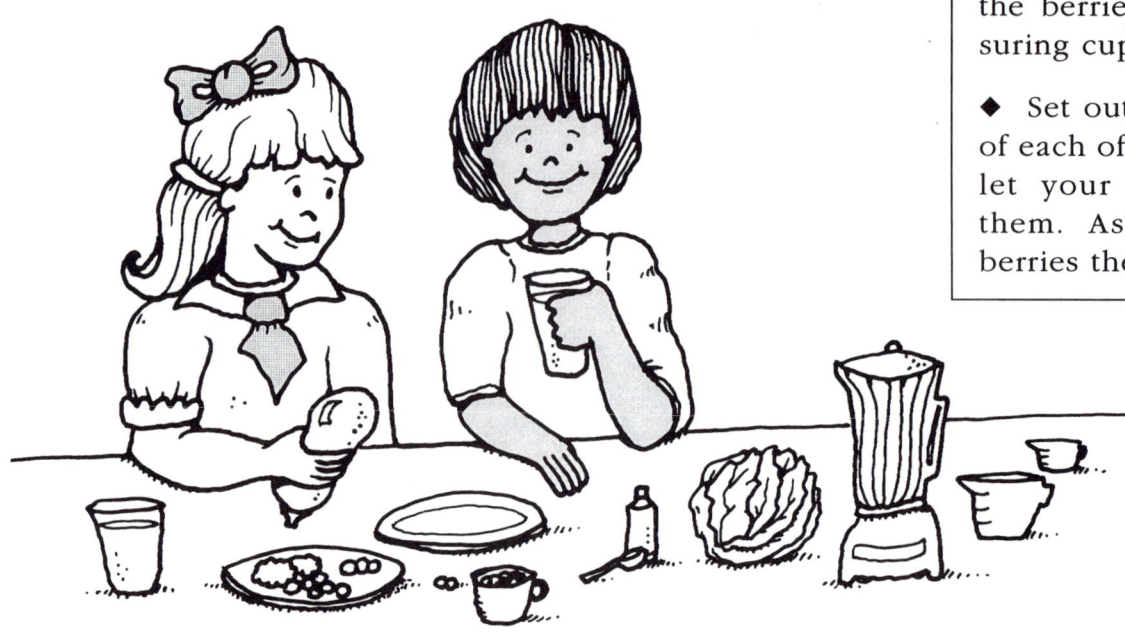

Discovering Colors

◆ Ask your children to name the color of the shake. Have them name other purple objects they know.

◆ Set out a banana, some raspberries, some blueberries, an orange, and a green apple. Ask your children to guess which two kinds of fruits were used in the shake to make the color purple.

◆ Set out purple-colored foods such as plums, grapes, grape juice, red cabbage, and eggplant. Let your children name the foods and, if desired, try some of each.

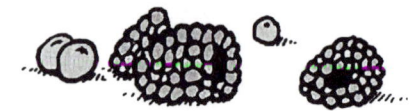

Creamy Alphabet Soup

1 cup alphabet-shaped pasta
3 cups chicken broth
½ cup chopped celery
¼ cup chopped onion
1 cup whole green beans
½ cup sliced carrots
1 bay leaf
1 cup milk

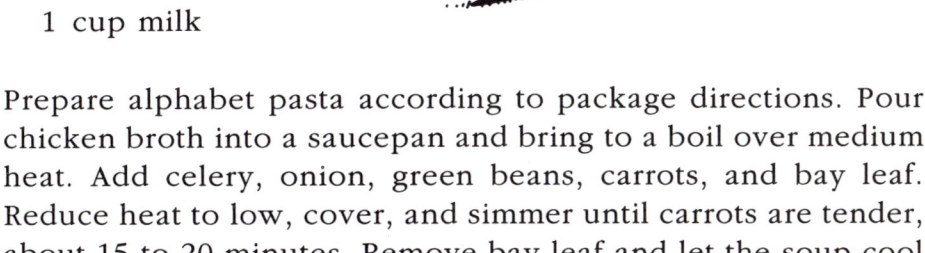

Prepare alphabet pasta according to package directions. Pour chicken broth into a saucepan and bring to a boil over medium heat. Add celery, onion, green beans, carrots, and bay leaf. Reduce heat to low, cover, and simmer until carrots are tender, about 15 to 20 minutes. Remove bay leaf and let the soup cool for 5 to 10 minutes. Add cooked pasta and stir in milk. Serve immediately. Makes ten ½-cup servings.

Cooking Skills

◆ Let your children compare some dried alphabet noodles to the cooked ones.

◆ Have your children help clean and prepare the vegetables.

◆ Let your children help measure the ingredients.

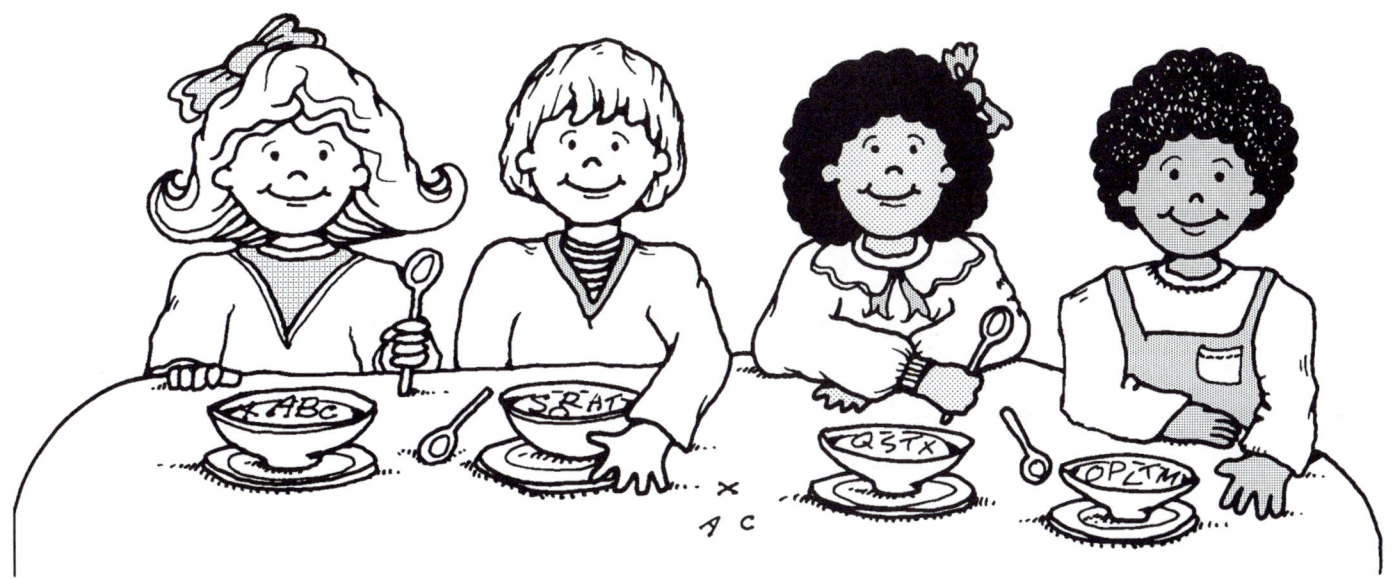

Discovering Letters

◆ Have your children find letters that they recognize, or letters in their names, in their Creamy Alphabet Soup.

◆ Name a letter and ask your children to try to find it in their soup.

◆ Sing "The ABC Song" with your children before they eat their soup.

◆ Ask your children to look for letters around the room.

◆ Show your children the containers the ingredients came in. Ask them to name any letters they recognize on the containers.

Alphabet Breadsticks

1 package active dry yeast
1½ cups warm water (110°F)
1 tablespoon honey
2 cups all-purpose flour
2 cups whole-wheat flour
　Melted butter or margarine
　Garlic salt, seasoning salt, or onion salt

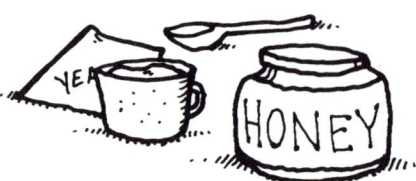

Place yeast in a large bowl. Add warm water and honey and stir. Let the mixture sit for a few minutes until bubbly. Stir in all-purpose flour. Add whole-wheat flour, ½ cup at a time. Mix thoroughly after each addition of flour, using a heavy wooden spoon or your hands. Dust additional flour over a smooth surface and turn the dough onto it. Knead the dough for 10 minutes. Grease a baking sheet. Cut the dough into quarters, then cut each quarter into 8 pieces. Roll each piece of dough until it is 10 inches long, place it on the baking sheet, and form it into the shape of a letter. Brush the letters with melted butter and lightly sprinkle with one of the salts. Let rise in a warm, draft-free place for 15 minutes. Bake at 400°F for 15 minutes. Makes 32 Alphabet Breadsticks.

Cooking Skills

◆ Let your children help measure and mix together the ingredients.

◆ Have your children take turns kneading the dough.

◆ Have your children help divide the dough. Let them count the pieces.

◆ Let your children roll out the dough and form it into letters or other shapes.

◆ Help your children use a pastry brush to gently brush butter on the breadsticks.

◆ Let your children take turns lightly sprinkling the seasoned salts on the breadsticks.

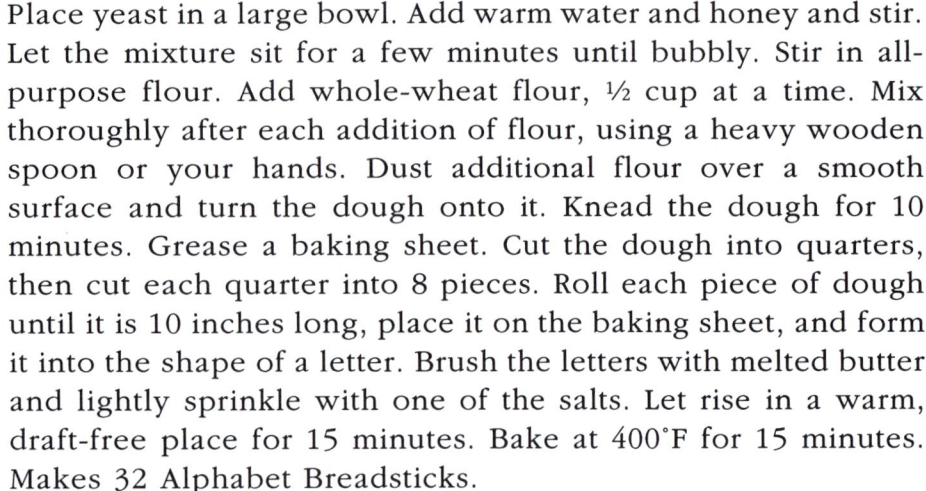

Discovering Letters

◆ Place the Alphabet Breadsticks on a tray and have your children name the letters.

◆ Let each child select an Alphabet Breadstick from a tray and name the letter.

◆ Make Alphabet Breadsticks using the beginning letters of your children's names. Have each child select the letter that begins his or her name.

◆ Use the Alphabet Breadsticks to spell out simple words.

◆ Make pairs of letters. Place them on a serving tray and let your children find the pairs.

Raisin Letters

1 package (8 ounces) cream cheese, softened
14 rice cakes
¾ cup raisins

Spread cream cheese on rice cakes. Place each rice cake on a plate. Use raisins to make letters on the rice cakes. Serves 14.

Variations: Instead of cream cheese, use 1 cup Yogurt Cheese (recipe on page 30). Or replace raisins with small pieces of fresh fruit such as oranges, peaches, or grapes. Or put raisin letters on small bowls of yogurt, scoops of cottage cheese, or slices of toast spread with peanut butter.

Cooking Skills

◆ Have your children spread the cheese on the rice cakes.

◆ Let your children put each rice cake on a plate.

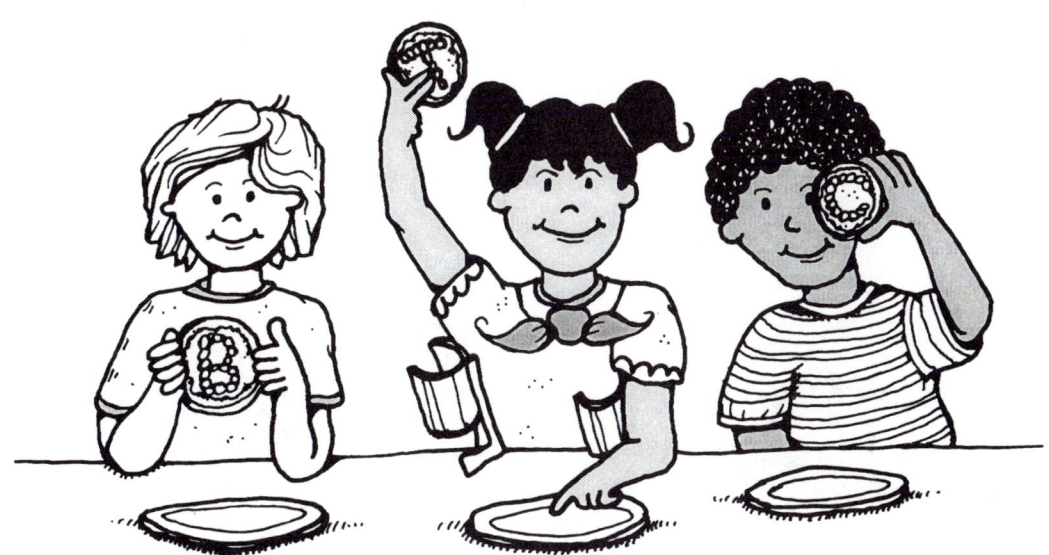

Discovering Letters

◆ Give each child a prepared rice cake without a letter on it. Have your children tell you the letters they want on their rice cakes.

◆ Select three letters. Decorate each rice cake with one of those letters. Let your children group together the rice cakes with the same letters on them. Then let the children choose which ones they want to eat.

◆ Put a different letter on each rice cake. Set them out on plates. Name the letters and let your children select the rice cakes with those letters on them. Or let your children select the rice cakes, naming the letters as they do so.

◆ Ask your children to name the letters on their rice cakes.

Sandwich Cut-Ups

Make a peanut-butter filling for sandwiches by combining peanut butter with a small amount of one or more of these ingredients: mashed bananas, chopped raisins or dates, applesauce, shredded coconut, or grated carrot. Spread the peanut-butter filling on slices of bread. Put the sandwiches together. Cut the sandwiches in a variety of ways such as in halves, quarters, triangles, and puzzle shapes. Place a whole sandwich on a plate for each child.

Hint: Partially freeze the bread slices ahead of time to make it easier to spread peanut butter on them. Be sure to allow about 15 minutes for the bread to thaw before eating.

Cooking Skills

◆ Let your children help mix together the ingredients for the peanut-butter filling.

◆ Have your children spread the peanut-butter filling on slices of partially frozen bread.

◆ Have your children tell you how they want their sandwiches cut.

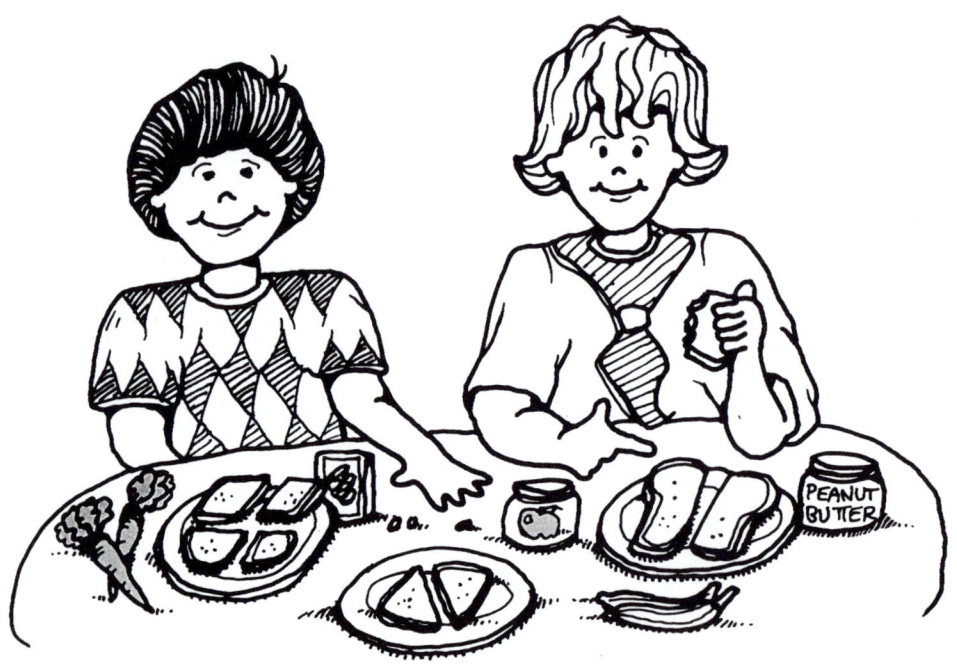

Discovering Math

◆ Have your children count the number of pieces in their sandwiches.

◆ Let your children move the pieces of their sandwiches around and then put them back.

◆ Talk about wholes, halves, and quarters. Ask your children to show you whole sandwiches, half sandwiches, and quarter sandwiches.

Counting Snack

For each child, set out a 6-cup muffin tin. Fill each cup of the muffin tin with a different number of food items. For example, you could put in 1 apple slice, 2 crackers, 3 cheese cubes, 4 grapes, 5 pretzels, and 6 cereal pieces.

Variation: Instead of using a muffin tin for each child, remove and discard the lid of an egg carton. Cut the bottom of the egg carton in half widthwise to make two units with six egg cups each. Use one of the egg-carton halves in place of a muffin tin.

Cooking Skills

◆ Have your children help you prepare the food for putting in the muffin cups.

◆ Let your children put paper baking cups in each of the muffin cups before putting in the food items.

◆ Have one of your children pass out a muffin tin to each child.

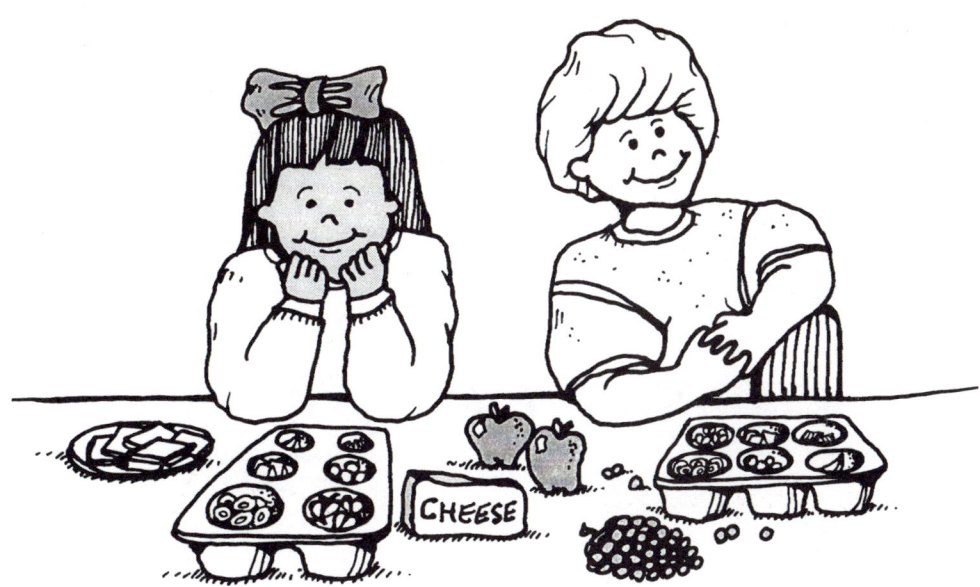

Discovering Math

◆ Have your children count the number of cups in their muffin tins.

◆ Ask your children to point to the muffin cup that has three items in it, five items in it, and so on.

◆ Let each child select one of the cups in his or her muffin tin and count the number of items in it.

◆ Ask your children to tell you how many of a particular food item they have.

◆ Set out the food items and give your children directions for filling their own muffin tins, such as these: "Put one apple slice in one muffin cup. Put two crackers in one muffin cup."

Number Mix

¼ cup *O*-shaped cereal pieces
1 cup square-shaped cereal pieces
2 cups popcorn
2 cups melba crackers
3 cups pretzel twists

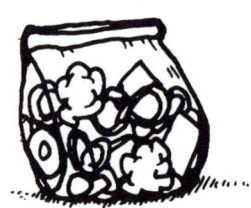

Put a different number (from 1 to 10) of each ingredient into a resealable plastic bag. Seal the bag and shake it to mix up the ingredients. Repeat for each bag. Makes about 12 bags of Number Mix.

Cooking Skills

◆ Have your children place each ingredient in a separate serving bowl.

◆ Let one of your children pass out a resealable bag to each child.

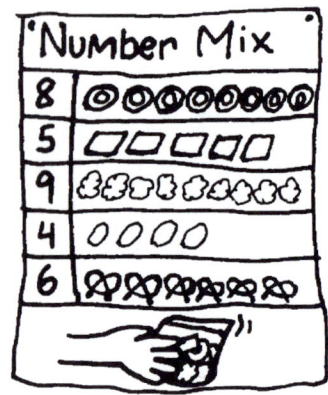

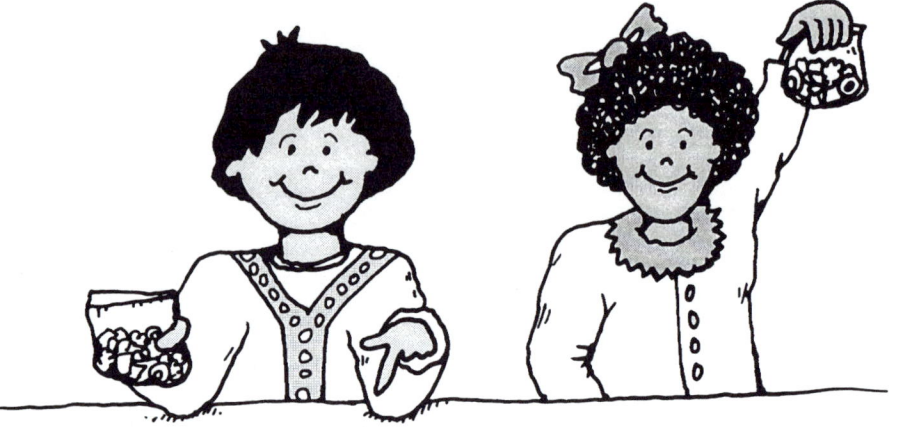

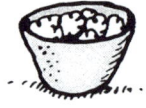 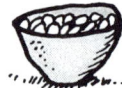 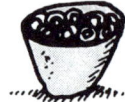 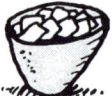 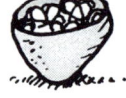

Discovering Math

◆ Have your children look at the ingredients in their Number Mix bags. Ask them to guess which item they have the most of and which one they have the least of.

◆ Ask your children to take all of one particular item out of their bags and count them.

◆ Make up a recipe chart that specifies the number of each ingredient that should go in each of your children's resealable bags. Then let your children "read" the chart, count out the items, and fill the bags.

◆ Let your children make their own Number Mix recipes. Have each child select a number between 1 and 5. Then have the child put that number of each ingredient in his or her bag.

◆ Before passing out prepared bags of Number Mix, have your children count the number of bags and the number of children. Ask them if there will be any extra bags. If so, can they tell you how many?

◆ Have your children carefully empty their bags onto napkins and sort the ingredients into piles before eating them.

Peanut Butter Playdough

¾ cup natural-style peanut butter
¾ cup toasted wheat germ
¼ cup honey
¼ cup powdered milk
  Raisins, nuts, sunflower seeds, coconut, etc., for decoration

Put peanut butter, wheat germ, honey, and powdered milk in a small bowl and mix them together thoroughly. Shape the playdough as desired. Set out raisins, nuts, sunflower seeds, coconut, etc., for decorating the dough. Makes 6 servings, 3 tablespoons each.

Single Serving—Combine 2 tablespoons peanut butter, 2 tablespoons toasted wheat germ, 2 teaspoons honey, and 2 teaspoons powered milk.

Hint: To save money, purchase raw wheat germ instead of toasted, and toast it yourself in a dry, hot skillet.

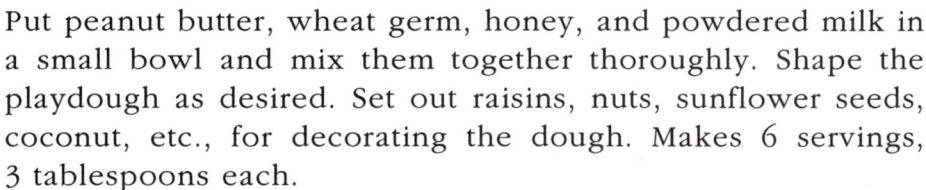

Cooking Skills

◆ Let your children help measure and mix together the ingredients for the playdough.

◆ Have your children put the items for decorating the playdough in separate bowls.

◆ Make a recipe chart for the single serving of Peanut Butter Playdough. Let your children measure and mix their own.

Discovering Math

◆ Let your children shape their pieces of playdough as desired. Then have each of them put four raisins, two peanuts, six sunflower seeds, etc., on their shapes.

◆ Have your children pat their playdough into circles. Give them table knives and help them cut their circles into halves and quarters.

◆ Give each of your children a piece of the Peanut Butter Playdough. Have them form the playdough into two balls, three balls, and so on.

Number Rolls

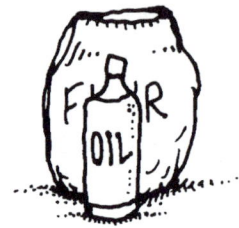

1 ½ cups all-purpose flour
1 ½ teaspoons salt
   ½ package active dry yeast (1 ⅛ teaspoons)
   1 tablespoon vegetable oil
   2 tablespoons honey
   1 cup plus 2 tablespoons warm water (110°F)
1 ½ cups whole-wheat flour

In a large bowl, mix all-purpose flour, salt, and yeast together. Add oil and honey, then stir in warm water. Add whole-wheat flour, a little at a time, mixing with a heavy wooden spoon or your hands. Knead the dough on a floured surface for 5 minutes, until the dough is smooth and satiny. Clean and oil the mixing bowl. Put the dough in the bowl and turn it to grease the top. Cover the bowl with clear-plastic wrap and put it in the refrigerator. Allow the dough to rise in the refrigerator for at least 2 hours, but no more than 48 hours.

Take the dough out of the refrigerator and knead for 1 to 2 minutes. Cut the dough into 16 pieces. Shape each piece into a ball and place them in a greased 9-inch round pan. Cover the pan with a damp cloth and let the dough rise for about 2 hours, or until doubled in size, in a warm, draft-free place. (An oven heated to 90°F to 100°F works well.) Bake at 375°F for 20 to 25 minutes, or until lightly browned. Makes 16 rolls.

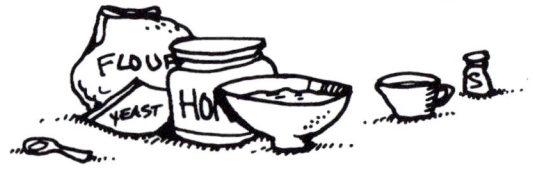

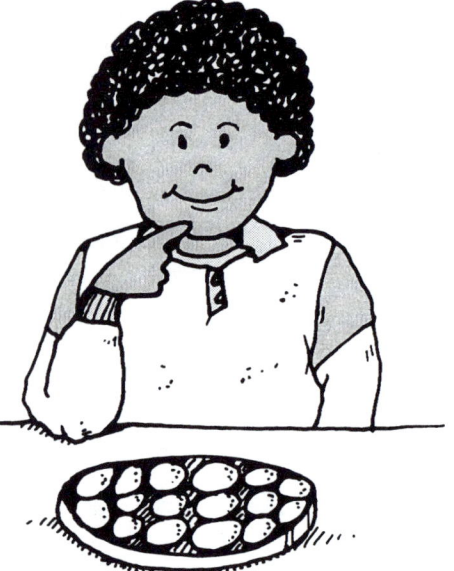

Cooking Skills

◆ Have your children help measure and mix together the ingredients.

◆ Let your children take turns kneading the dough.

◆ Give your children the pieces of dough and have them roll the dough into balls.

◆ Let your children arrange the balls of dough in the greased pan.

Discovering Math

◆ Let your children help divide the dough into 16 pieces. Divide it in half to make two pieces, divide those pieces in half again to make four pieces, and so on.

◆ Have your children divide their rolls in half before eating them.

◆ Show your children the pan of rolls. Ask them to guess how many rolls are in the pan. Then take the rolls out of the pan and separate them. Let your children count the rolls.

Pizza Pie

1 teaspoon active dry yeast
½ cup lukewarm water (105°F)
¼ teaspoon salt
2 tablespoons olive oil, divided
1 ¼ cups all-purpose flour
½ cup pizza sauce or tomato sauce
2 cups shredded cheese
    Pizza toppings such as Canadian bacon, sausage, pineapple, olives, and mushrooms

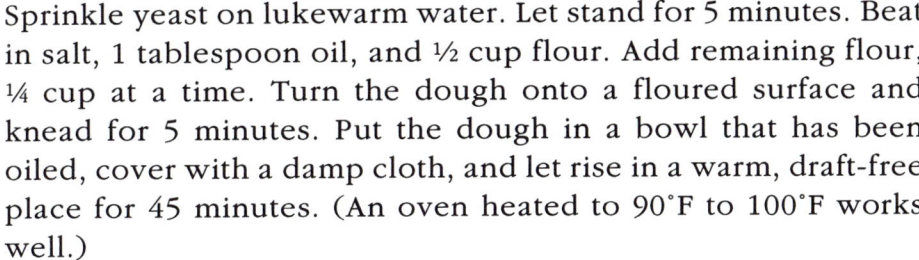

Sprinkle yeast on lukewarm water. Let stand for 5 minutes. Beat in salt, 1 tablespoon oil, and ½ cup flour. Add remaining flour, ¼ cup at a time. Turn the dough onto a floured surface and knead for 5 minutes. Put the dough in a bowl that has been oiled, cover with a damp cloth, and let rise in a warm, draft-free place for 45 minutes. (An oven heated to 90°F to 100°F works well.)

Grease a 12-inch pizza pan. Punch the dough down and knead 2 minutes. Roll out the dough to fit in the pan and press into place. Brush with remaining olive oil, spread on sauce, and sprinkle on cheese and desired toppings. Bake at 500°F for 10 to 12 minutes, until crust is cooked. Allow the pizza to cool for 10 minutes before cutting it into the desired number of slices. Makes one 12-inch pizza.

Cooking Skills

◆ Have your children help measure and mix together the ingredients for the pizza dough.

◆ Let your children take turns kneading the dough.

◆ Let your children help shred the cheese and prepare the toppings.

◆ Have your children spread the sauce on top of the pizza crust and arrange the toppings.

◆ Let your children select which toppings they want on their pizza.

Discovering Math

◆ Begin serving the pizza. Have your children watch as each part of the pizza is removed. Point out when a quarter of the pizza is gone, when half of it is gone, and so on.

◆ Let your children look at their slices of pizza. Ask them if they can find toppings that are whole pieces and toppings that are just parts of whole pieces.

◆ Make two or three pizzas. Cut each pizza into a different number of pieces (quarters, sixths, eighths). Show your children a slice from each pizza. Ask them which one is biggest, which one is smallest.

◆ Show your children the pizza. Have them count the number of slices.

Date Balls

8 ounces (1 ½ cups) chopped dates
4 ounces (½ cup) water
1 ounce (¼ cup) finely chopped walnuts
4 ounces (3 cups) wheat-flake cereal, crushed
    Shredded coconut

Place dates and water in a medium-sized saucepan and bring to a boil. Cover and simmer for 5 minutes, or until dates are soft. Remove dates from heat (do not drain) and stir in walnuts and crushed cereal. Allow to cool slightly. Form tablespoonfuls of the date mixture into balls. Roll the balls in coconut and refrigerate until firm. Makes about 32 Date Balls.

Cooking Skills

◆ Put the wheat flakes in a resealable plastic bag, squeeze out all the air, seal the bag, and let your children crush the wheat flakes by rolling a rolling pin over the bag.

◆ Let your children roll the Date Balls in the shredded coconut.

◆ Instead of mixing the ingredients together in the saucepan, put them in a large bowl and let your children use their hands to mix them together.

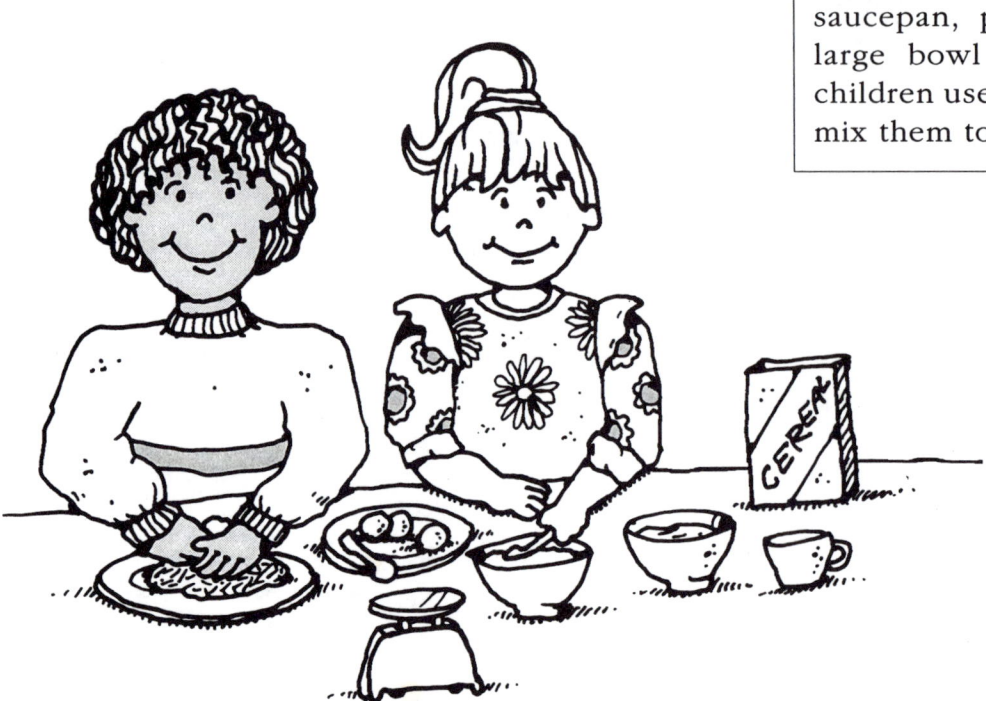

Discovering Math

◆ Show your children a tablespoon and let them measure out the date mixture to roll.

◆ Have your children count the number of Date Balls made.

◆ Prepare this recipe with your children using a kitchen scale to weigh the ingredients rather than using measuring cups.

Popcorn

Place popcorn kernels in an air popper or heavy, oiled pan and pop them. Toss the hot popcorn with melted butter or margarine in a large bowl. Place small amounts of the popcorn in resealable plastic bags. Sprinkle the popcorn in each bag with one of the following toppings: Parmesan cheese, seasoning salt, cinnamon sugar, or powdered ranch dressing mix. Seal the bags and shake to combine popcorn and toppings.

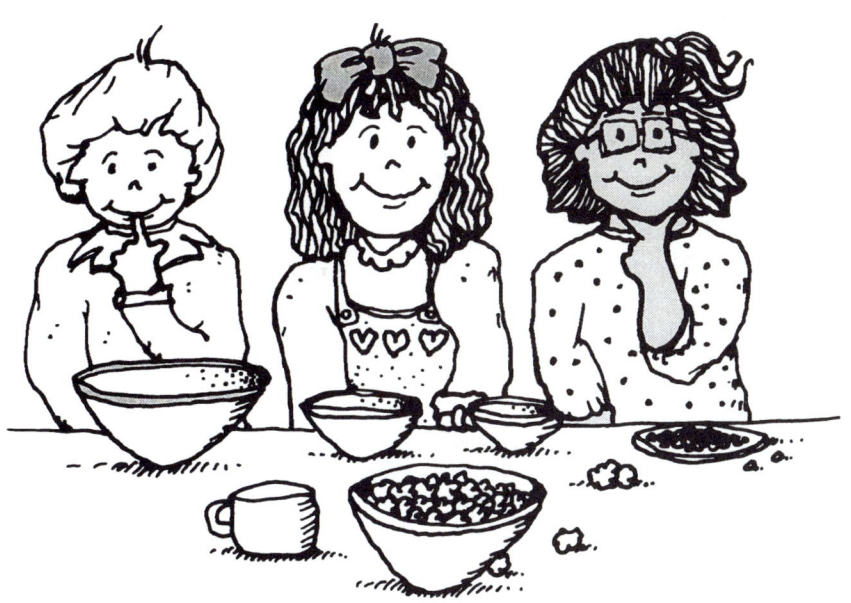

Cooking Skills

◆ If you use a hot-air popcorn popper, let your children fill the popper with popcorn and put butter or margarine in the cup for melting.

◆ Let your children use spoons to mix the popcorn with the butter or margarine and salt.

◆ Set out several shakers filled with the popcorn toppings. Let your children sprinkle small amounts of the toppings of their choice in their bags of popcorn. Seal the bags, then let the children shake them to mix the popcorn and toppings.

Discovering Science

◆ Let your children watch while you make popcorn in a variety of ways: in an air popper, in a pan on the stove, in the microwave, or in a Jiffy Pop-brand popper (available at grocery stores). Or let them watch popcorn being made in a commercial popping machine at a movie theater or a popcorn stand.

◆ Set out different sizes of bowls. Ask your children to arrange the bowls in order from that which will hold the most popcorn to that which will hold the least. Then fill the bowls with cups of popcorn to find out if they were right.

◆ Let your children measure out a particular amount of popcorn kernels, such as ¼ cup. Ask them to predict how much popped corn that amount will make. Then pop the kernels and measure the popcorn.

◆ Collect different varieties of popcorn kernels such as yellow, white, blue, and red (available at specialty-food stores and some supermarkets). Have your children predict what color the popped corn will be.

◆ Have your children compare a popcorn kernel with a piece of popped corn.

Butter

Make butter in any of the following ways. Add a small amount of salt to the finished butter, if desired. Serve with crackers or bread.

Shaking—Fill a baby food jar halfway with whipping cream and shake the jar until the butter forms a ball.

Mixing—Put 1 cup of whipping cream in a mixing bowl and beat on medium-high until the butter forms.

Blending—Put 1 cup of whipping cream in a blender container and blend until the butter separates from the liquid.

Rolling—Find a small container with a tight-fitting lid. Fill it halfway with whipping cream. Put the lid on the container and place it in a 13-ounce coffee can with a lid. Pack newspaper around the container, then put the lid on the coffee can. Roll the container back and forth (for at least 15 minutes), until butter is formed.

Hint: One quart (4 cups) of whipping cream yields 1½ cups butter and 1¾ cups buttermilk. If desired, use some of the butter and buttermilk to make Buttermilk Biscuits (recipe on page 41).

Cooking Skills

◆ Let your children help measure and pour the whipping cream into the various containers.

◆ Help your children shake some salt on the finished butter and stir it in.

◆ Let your children spread the butter on crackers or bread they have selected.

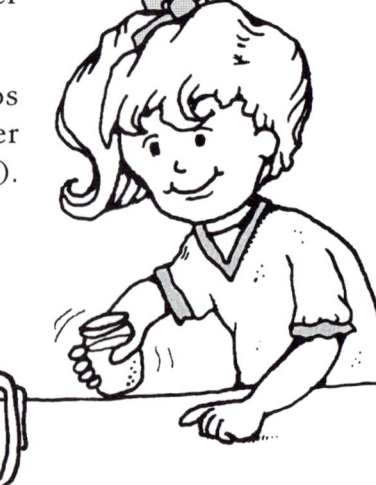

Discovering Science

◆ Show your children some whipping cream in a baby-food jar. Have them predict what will happen when you shake the jar. Stop to observe the changes in the whipping cream while you are shaking it. (It will take about 5 minutes for the butter to form.)

◆ Let your children compare some whipping cream with the butter and buttermilk that it forms after shaking.

◆ Have each of the different methods to make butter available to your children. Let them compare the time and results from each method.

Lemon Sherbet

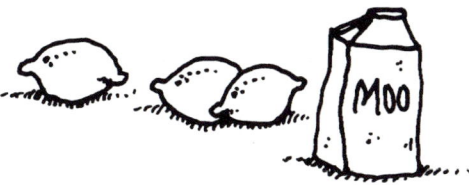

3 lemons
2 cups sugar
4 cups milk
1 cup whipping cream

Grate the rind of one of the lemons. Roll lemons back and forth several times while pressing on them firmly (this helps release the juice). Cut lemons in half and squeeze out the juice. Mix lemon rind, juice, and sugar together. Add milk and stir thoroughly. Use a mixer to whip the whipping cream until soft peaks form. Set aside.

Prepare an ice-cream freezer with ice and salt according to the manufacturer's directions. Pour the lemon mixture into the freezing can and, just before starting, stir in whipped cream. Process the mixture until it is the consistency of sherbet. Makes 4 cups.

Cooking Skills

◆ Let your children roll the lemons and then help you squeeze the juice out of them.

◆ Let your children help measure and mix together the ingredients.

◆ If possible, use a hand-cranked ice-cream maker and let your children take turns cranking the handle. (Be sure to have adult help available when the handle gets hard to turn.)

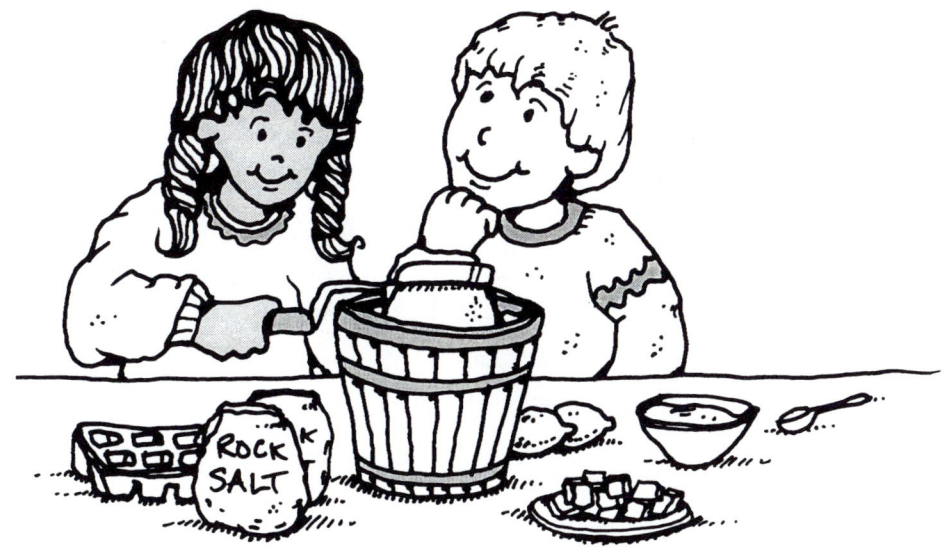

Discovering Science

◆ Ask your children to predict what will happen to the lemon mixture when it is put in the ice-cream freezer.

◆ Save a little bit of the lemon mixture. Let your children compare the liquid with the frozen sherbet.

◆ Ask your children to think of other foods they eat that are frozen.

◆ Put a few pieces of ice in two different bowls. Sprinkle rock salt on the ice in one bowl. Have your children observe the ice after 10 minutes.

Yogurt Cheese

Line a strainer with 2 layers of cheesecloth or a paper coffee filter. Place the strainer over a bowl. Spoon vanilla or fruit-flavored yogurt into the strainer. Fill a plastic bag with about 1 pound of dried beans or another heavy food. Place the plastic bag on top of the yogurt. (This helps squeeze the liquid out of the yogurt.) Put the yogurt in the refrigerator and allow it to drain for at least 30 minutes. (The longer it drains, the firmer the Yogurt Cheese will be.) Remove the Yogurt Cheese from the cheesecloth and store in an airtight container in the refrigerator. Spread the cheese on crackers, bagels, or toast. Four cups of yogurt makes 1½ cups of Yogurt Cheese.

Cooking Skills

◆ Let your children spoon the yogurt into the strainer.

◆ Set out several kinds of flavored yogurt. Let your children choose which kind to use to make the Yogurt Cheese.

◆ Have your children spread the Yogurt Cheese on crackers.

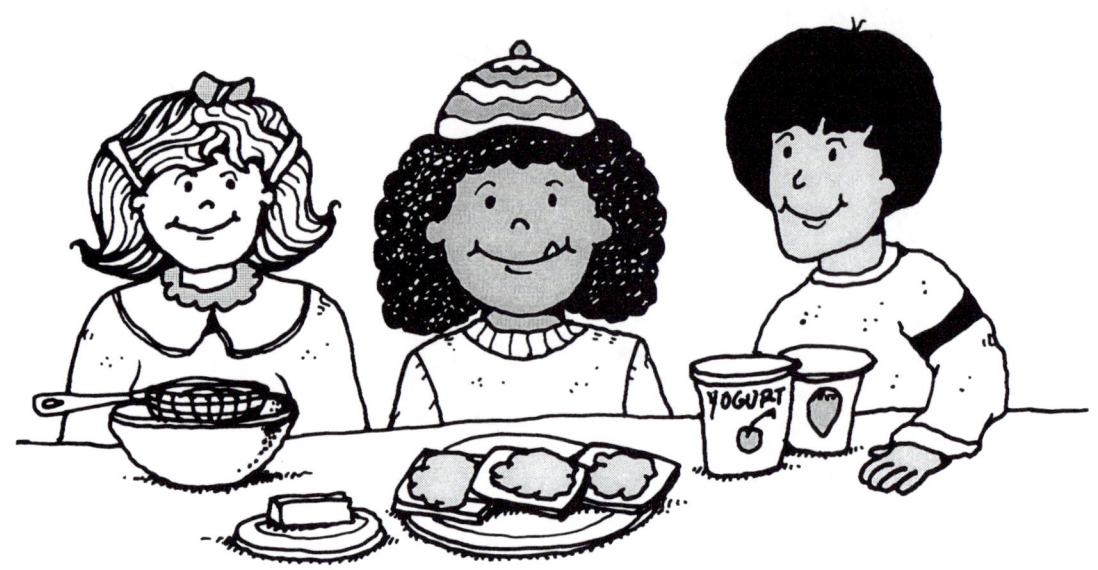

Discovering Science

◆ Just before placing the strainer setup in the refrigerator, show it to your children. Ask them to predict what will happen to the yogurt. When the Yogurt Cheese is ready, have them compare their predictions to what actually happened.

◆ Make two or three different flavors of Yogurt Cheese. Put a sample of each kind on a plate for each child. Have your children close their eyes, taste the cheeses, and try to guess which flavors they are.

◆ Show your children some regular yogurt and some Yogurt Cheese. Let them look at, smell, feel, and taste the yogurt and the Yogurt Cheese. Ask the children to tell you how they are alike and how they are different.

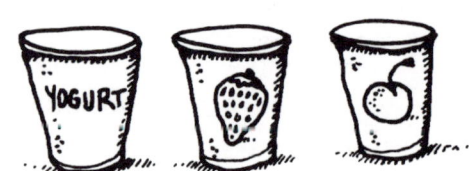

Bean Dip

1 cup pinto beans
8 cups water, divided
1 teaspoon garlic powder
½ teaspoon cumin
½ teaspoon oregano
2 teaspoons chili powder
¼ teaspoon salt
¼ cup plain yogurt
¼ cup shredded Cheddar cheese
Tortilla chips or vegetable sticks

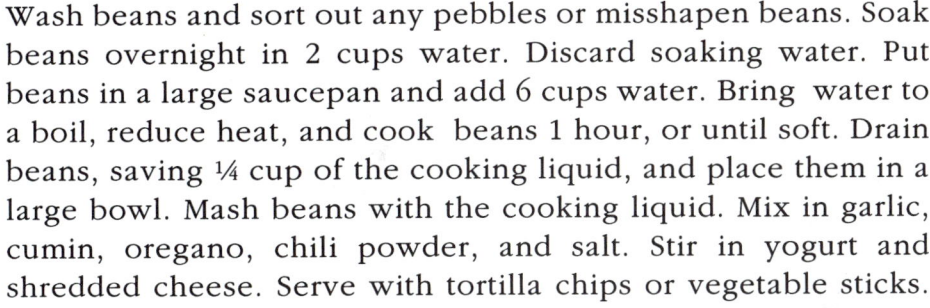

Wash beans and sort out any pebbles or misshapen beans. Soak beans overnight in 2 cups water. Discard soaking water. Put beans in a large saucepan and add 6 cups water. Bring water to a boil, reduce heat, and cook beans 1 hour, or until soft. Drain beans, saving ¼ cup of the cooking liquid, and place them in a large bowl. Mash beans with the cooking liquid. Mix in garlic, cumin, oregano, chili powder, and salt. Stir in yogurt and shredded cheese. Serve with tortilla chips or vegetable sticks. Makes 2¼ cups of dip.

Cooking Skills

◆ Let your children measure out the beans, then wash and sort them. Have them measure the water for soaking and cooking.

◆ Have your children use a potato masher to mash the beans.

◆ Have your children help measure out the remaining ingredients.

◆ Let your children help shred the cheese.

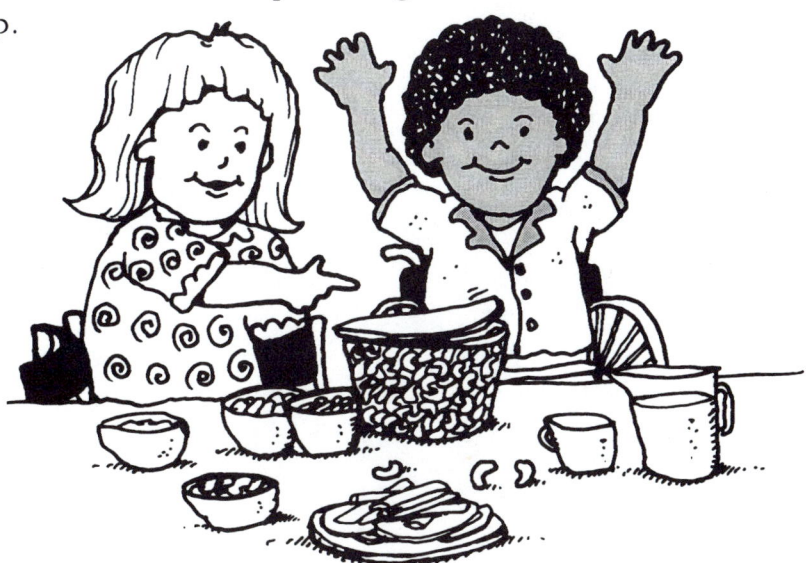

Discovering Science

◆ Find a small plastic container with a snap-on lid and fill it with dried beans. Add water up to the brim, then put on the lid. Show it to your children. Let the container sit overnight. In the morning, the beans will have absorbed the water and expanded enough to push the lid off.

◆ Let your children plant a few pinto beans. They should grow like regular bean seeds.

◆ Save a few beans from each stage of the cooking process: uncooked, soaked, cooked, and mashed. Show them to your children and have them compare the different beans.

Hot Cocoa

¼ cup unsweetened cocoa
½ cup sugar
   Dash of salt
⅓ cup hot water
4 cups milk
1 teaspoon vanilla extract
1 can (6 ½ ounces) whipped cream

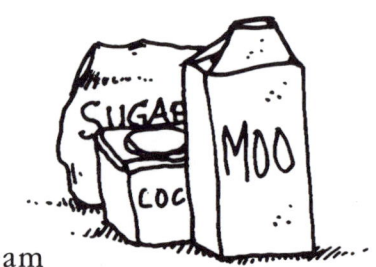

Mix cocoa, sugar, and salt together in a large saucepan. Stir in hot water. Bring to a boil over medium heat, stirring constantly. Continue stirring while the mixture boils for 2 minutes. Pour in milk. Stir until milk is heated. (Do not boil.) Remove from heat and add vanilla. Pour into mugs. Top with whipped cream. Makes nine ½-cup servings.

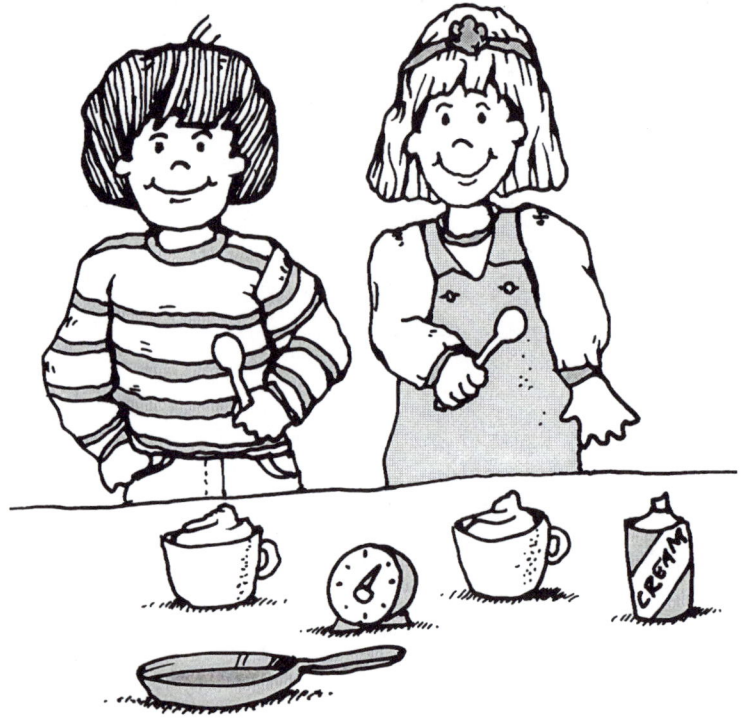

Cooking Skills

◆ Let your children help measure and mix together the dry ingredients.

◆ Have your children watch as you add the hot water to the cocoa mixture. Ask them to notice how the color changes.

◆ Show your children how to set a timer for 2 minutes. Let them watch and listen to the timer. Have them tell you when the time is up.

◆ Buy the milk in a quart carton. Show your children that the carton contains exactly 4 cups by pouring the milk into a measuring cup.

◆ Let your children "squirt" the whipped cream on their own mugs of cocoa.

Discovering Opposites

◆ Serve the cocoa with spoons. Let your children use the spoons to taste the cold whipped cream and the hot cocoa.

◆ Ask your children to name other hot foods and other cold foods that they eat.

◆ Have your children think of other things that are hot (sun, heater, oven, etc.) and other things that are cold (refrigerator, ice cube, snow, etc.).

Crunchy-Creamy Treats

2 tablespoons vegetable oil
2 tablespoons honey
¼ cup unsweetened apple juice
½ teaspoon vanilla extract
2 cups regular rolled oats
½ cup raw wheat germ
¼ cup chopped almonds
½ cup shredded coconut
    Plain, vanilla, or fruit-flavored yogurt

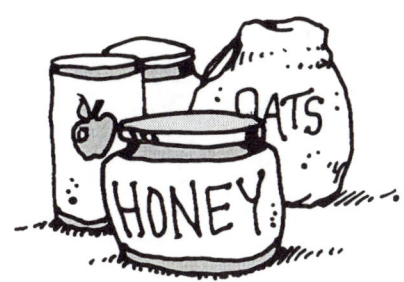

To make crunchy granola, mix oil, honey, apple juice, and vanilla in a small saucepan. Heat on low until honey is melted. In a 9-by-13-inch baking pan, mix together rolled oats, wheat germ, chopped almonds, and shredded coconut. Carefully pour in honey mixture and stir until thoroughly combined. Bake at 350°F for 30 minutes, stirring every 10 minutes. Cool. Makes 3 cups granola. Spoon yogurt into small bowls and sprinkle granola on top to make Crunchy-Creamy Treats.

Cooking Skills

◆ Let your children help measure and mix together the ingredients for the granola.

◆ Set out two or three different kinds of yogurt and let each child select which kind he or she would like.

◆ Let your children spoon small amounts of yogurt into bowls and sprinkle granola on top.

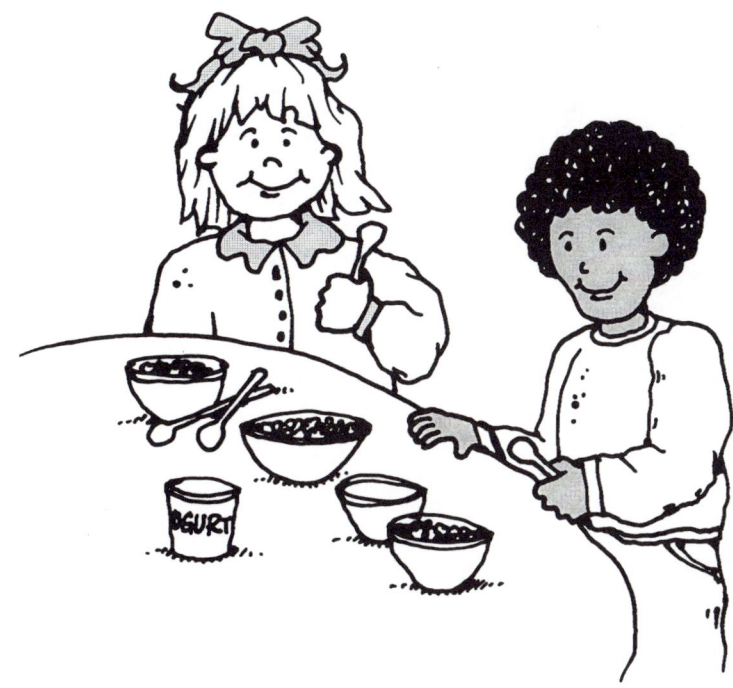

Discovering Opposites

◆ Let your children taste the creamy yogurt and the crunchy granola separately. Ask them to describe how each food feels in their mouths. Have them tell you which food is easiest to chew.

◆ Have your children name other foods they like that are crunchy or creamy.

Lemonade

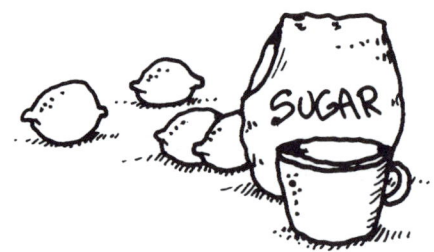

4 lemons
3 cups water
½ cup sugar
  Ice cubes
  Lemon slices

Roll lemons back and forth several times while pressing on them firmly (this helps to release the juice). Slice lemons in half and squeeze the juice out of them with a juicer or your hands. Put the juice in a pitcher. Add water and sugar to lemon juice, and stir. Place ice cubes in small cups and pour the lemonade over the ice. Garnish with lemon slices. Makes eight ½-cup servings.

Cooking Skills

◆ Let your children roll the lemons, then help you squeeze the juice out of them.

◆ Have your children measure the water and sugar, then stir the lemonade.

◆ Let your children put ice cubes in small cups. Then help them pour some lemonade into each cup.

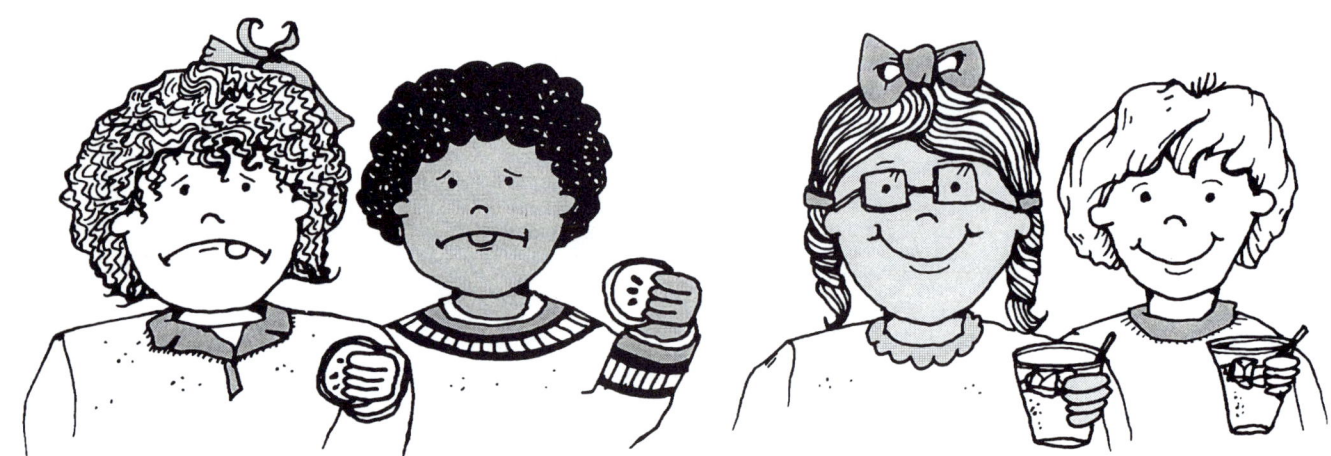

Discovering Opposites

◆ Have your children taste the lemon garnishes on their lemonades. Ask them to describe how the lemon tastes. Then have them taste their lemonade. Ask them to guess what is in the lemonade that makes it sweeter.

◆ Talk about the tastes of sour and sweet. Have your children name other foods that have the same tastes.

◆ Warm up some of the lemonade. Serve your children small amounts of warm and cold lemonade. Let them compare opposites in temperature.

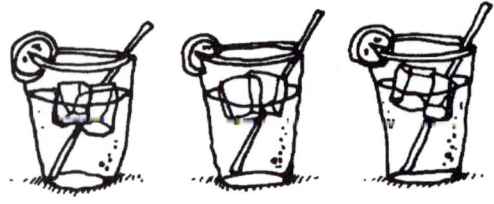

Toast Faces

Cut circles out of bread slices and toast them. (Use a variety of breads such as whole-wheat, sourdough, pumpernickel, and rye.) Save the left-over bread to feed the birds. Spread the toast circles with cream cheese, peanut butter, or Yogurt Cheese (recipe on page 30). Decorate the toast circles with grated carrot, alfalfa sprouts, olive slices, raisins, frozen blueberries, and O-shaped cereal pieces as desired to make faces.

Cooking Skills

◆ Let your children use a biscuit cutter or an inverted glass to cut circles out of the bread slices.

◆ Have your children spread the peanut butter, cream cheese, or Yogurt Cheese on the toast circles.

◆ Let your children help prepare and put in bowls the foods used for decorating the toast circles.

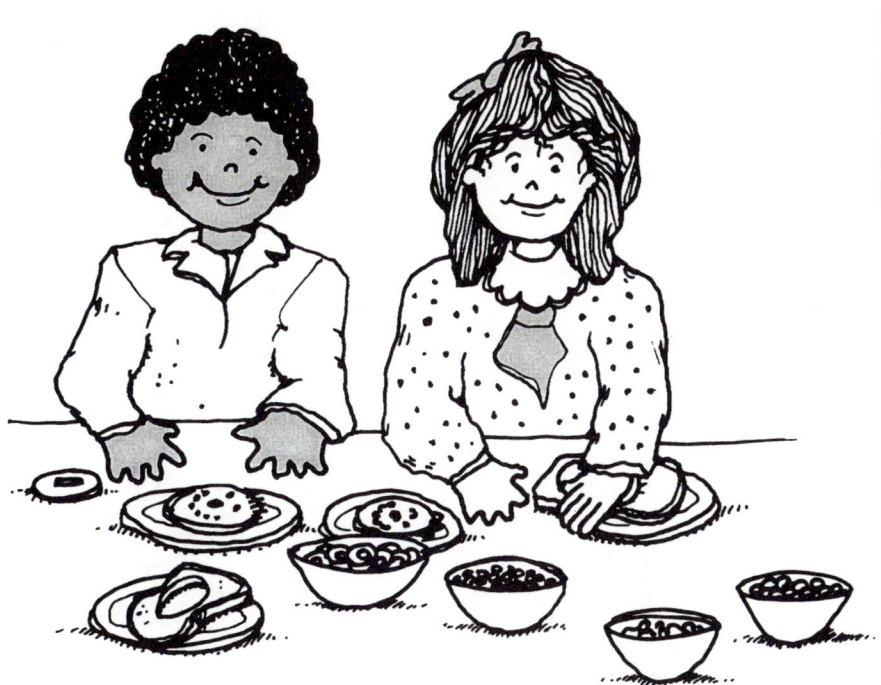

Developing Self-Esteem

◆ Set out bowls of grated carrot, alfalfa sprouts, olive slices, raisins, frozen blueberries, and O-shaped cereal pieces. Let each child select one of the prepared toast circles and have him or her use the food decorations to make a "self-portrait."

◆ Give your children the prepared toast circles and, instead of making self-portraits, let them decorate the circles as desired.

◆ Make a display of your children's decorated toast circles. Let them look at each other's creations and tell one another what they like about them.

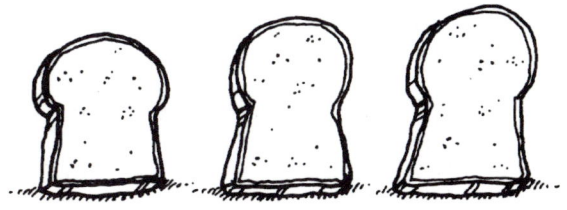

Baked Fruit

Fruit:

Apples

Apricots

Peaches

Pears

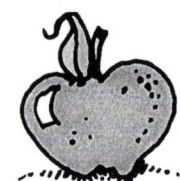

Fillings:

All-fruit spread

Chopped dates

Chopped nuts

Raisins

Sunflower seeds

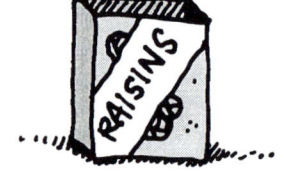

Toppings:

Chopped nuts

Granola

Toasted wheat germ

Cinnamon

Ground cloves

Nutmeg

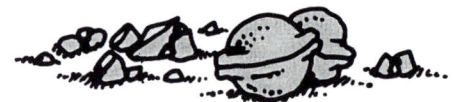

For each child, core one of the fruits from the list above. Place fruit in a baking dish. Add enough water to the dish to cover the bottom. Fill the centers of the fruit with any combination of fillings. Then sprinkle one or more of the toppings on fruit. Bake at 350°F for 20 to 35 minutes, or until fruit is soft. Serve warm.

Cooking Skills

◆ Let your children wash the fruit.

◆ Have your children put each filling and topping in a separate bowl.

◆ Let your children arrange the fruit in the baking pan.

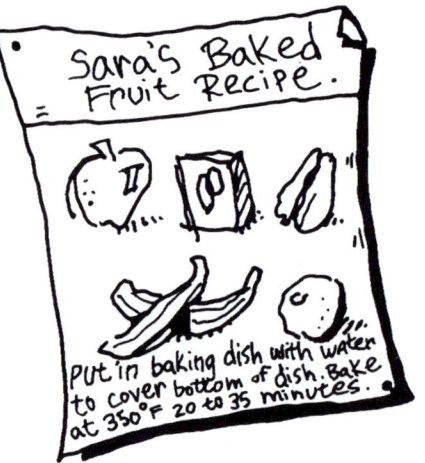

Developing Self-Esteem

◆ Set out the cored fruits, fillings, and toppings. Let each child prepare one of the fruits with the fillings and toppings he or she likes best.

◆ Lead your children in a discussion of likes and dislikes. Point out that each one of them is a unique person with likes and dislikes of his or her own.

◆ If your children prepare their own fruit, help them make recipe cards for their creations. On a plain white piece of paper write "_____'s Baked Fruit Recipe" at the top. At the bottom write "Put in baking dish with water to cover bottom of dish. Bake at 350°F for 20 to 35 minutes." Make a photocopy of this paper for each child. Then have your children draw pictures on their papers of the fruit, fillings, and toppings they used.

Tortilla Roll-Ups

Warm flour tortillas by wrapping a stack of them in damp paper towels then covering them with aluminum foil. Place the wrapped tortillas in a 300°F oven for 3 to 5 minutes. Set out a variety of fillings for the tortillas such as cooked ground turkey, Bean Dip (recipe on page 31), shredded cheese, chopped tomatoes, shredded lettuce, avocado slices, sliced olives, chopped onions, salsa, and sour cream or plain yogurt. Put each warmed-up tortilla on a plate, fill it with the desired toppings, and roll it up "burrito style."

Cooking Skills

◆ Let your children wrap the tortillas in the damp paper towels and aluminum foil.

◆ Have your children help prepare the fillings. Let them put each filling in a different bowl.

◆ Set out the plates and the tortillas. Have your children put one tortilla on each plate. Then let one or two of them pass out the plates.

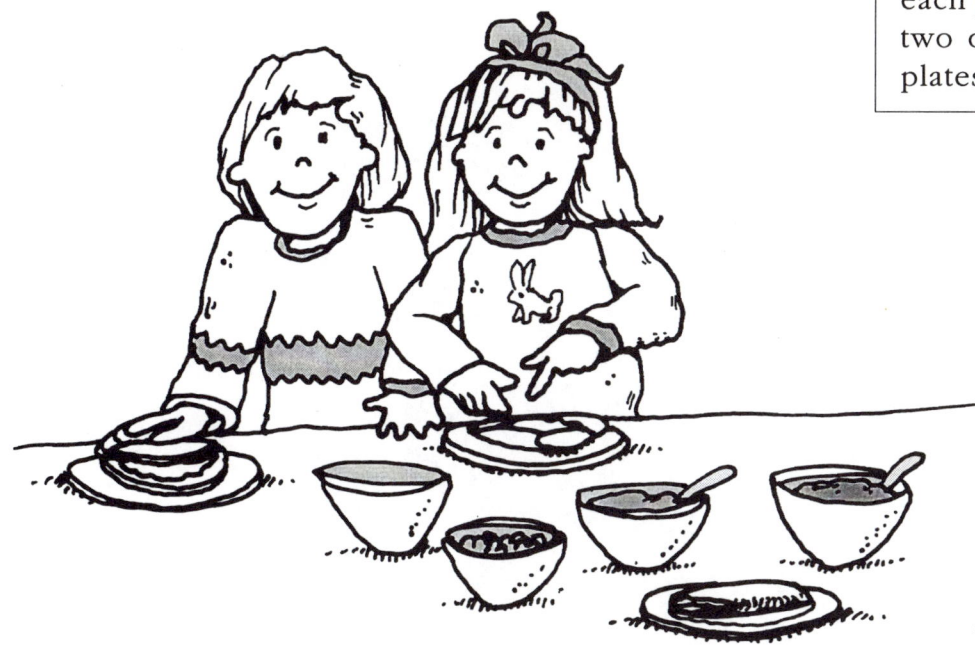

Developing Self-Esteem

◆ Give each of your children a plate with a tortilla. Let your children fill their tortillas with the kind and amount of fillings they want.

◆ Show your children how to roll up a tortilla. Ask them if they can think of any other ways to roll it up. Then let them decide how they will roll up their tortillas.

◆ Have your children talk about what fillings they put in their tortillas. Let them make up names for their tortillas. For example, if a tortilla had only tomatoes, lettuce, and avocado, it might be called a "garden tortilla."

Potato Sculpture

4 potatoes
2 tablespoons butter or margarine
2 tablespoons milk
1 teaspoon salt
1 egg white, lightly beaten

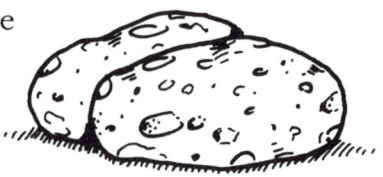

Peel potatoes and cut in quarters. Place in a large pan, cover with water, and bring to a boil. Reduce heat and simmer 12 to 15 minutes. Drain. Mash potatoes, then stir in butter, milk, and salt until smooth. Put potatoes in a greased 9-inch round or square baking pan. Use spoons, forks, or craft sticks to sculpt potatoes. Brush sculpted potatoes with egg white. Broil for 5 minutes, or until shiny and lightly browned. Allow to cool slightly before serving. Makes 2 cups mashed potatoes.

Cooking Skills

◆ Let your children count and wash the potatoes for you to peel.

◆ Have your children help measure the butter, milk, and salt.

◆ Let your children watch while you separate the egg white from the egg yolk. Give them a whisk to lightly beat the egg white.

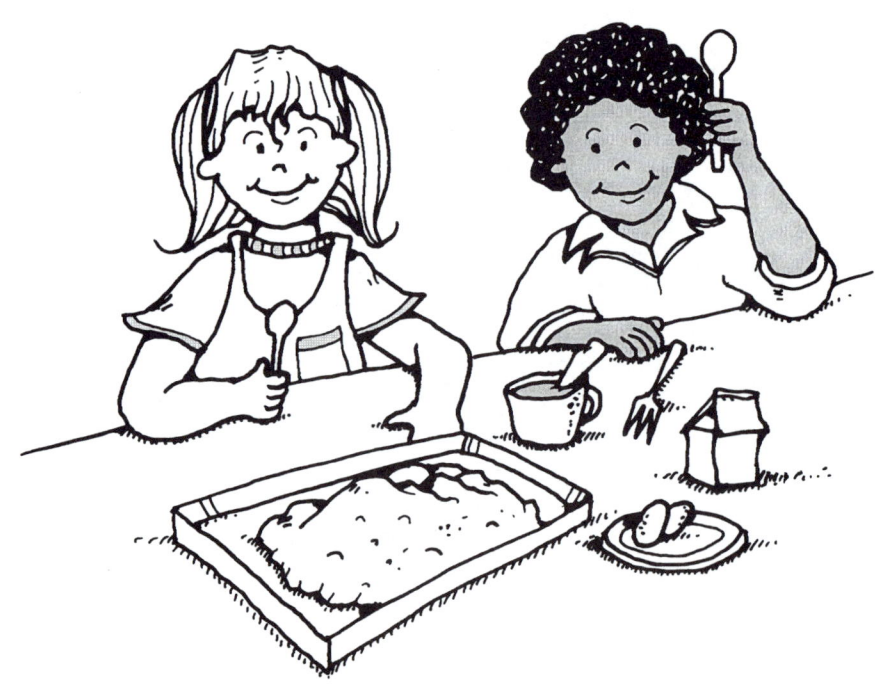

Developing Cooperation Skills

◆ Let your children take turns brushing their finished sculptures with the beaten egg white.

◆ Divide your children into groups of two to four. Make a pan of potatoes for each group. Let your children work together to sculpt the potatoes.

◆ Let each group of children work together to make the potatoes. Give them the cooked potatoes, slightly cooled, and premeasured butter, milk, and salt. Let them mash the potatoes, then put them into the pans for sculpting.

Crispy Bars

3 tablespoons peanut butter, at room temperature
4 to 6 tablespoons honey or pure maple syrup
1 cup chopped dates, raisins, or currants
½ cup sunflower seeds
2 cups crispy rice cereal

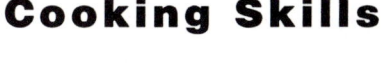

Grease an 8-inch square baking pan. Place all ingredients in a large bowl and mix well with your hands. Press the cereal mixture into the greased pan and freeze. Cut into squares. Eat the squares frozen or allow to thaw slightly. Makes sixteen 2-inch squares.

Cooking Skills

◆ Let your children help measure out the ingredients.

◆ Offer your children the choices in the list of ingredients (honey or maple syrup; dates, raisins, or currants). Let them select which ingredient (or combination of ingredients) they would like.

◆ Have your children place the cut squares on a serving platter. Let one or two of them pass out the squares to the other children.

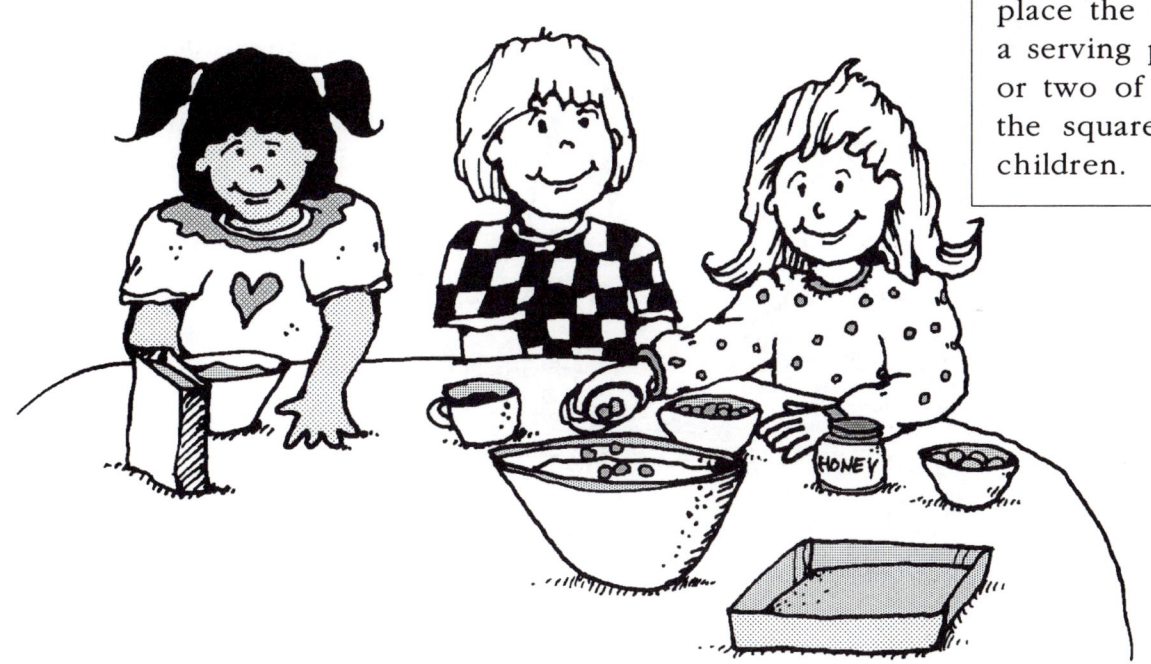

Developing Cooperation Skills

◆ Divide all of the ingredients among your children. Have each child put his or her ingredient in the bowl.

◆ Let your children work together to press the mixture into the greased pan.

◆ Put the ingredients in the mixing bowl and place it on a low table. Ask four of your children to stand around the bowl and each put one hand into it. Encourage them to work together to mix up the ingredients.

Vegetable Soup

Put vegetable, chicken, or beef broth in a large pan and bring to a boil. Prepare a variety of vegetables such as carrots, celery, potatoes, onions, bell peppers, peas, corn, mushrooms, and cabbage. Cut the vegetables into bite-size pieces. Place the vegetables in the boiling broth, turn down the heat, and simmer until the vegetables are tender, 10 to 15 minutes. Let the soup cool slightly before serving.

Cooking Skills

◆ Let your children choose the kind of broth they would like: vegetable, chicken, or beef. If you make the broth from bouillon, have them watch the bouillon powder or cubes dissolve in the hot water.

◆ Have your children wash and help prepare the vegetables.

◆ Put the finished soup in a soup tureen. Let your children take turns using a ladle to spoon the soup into bowls.

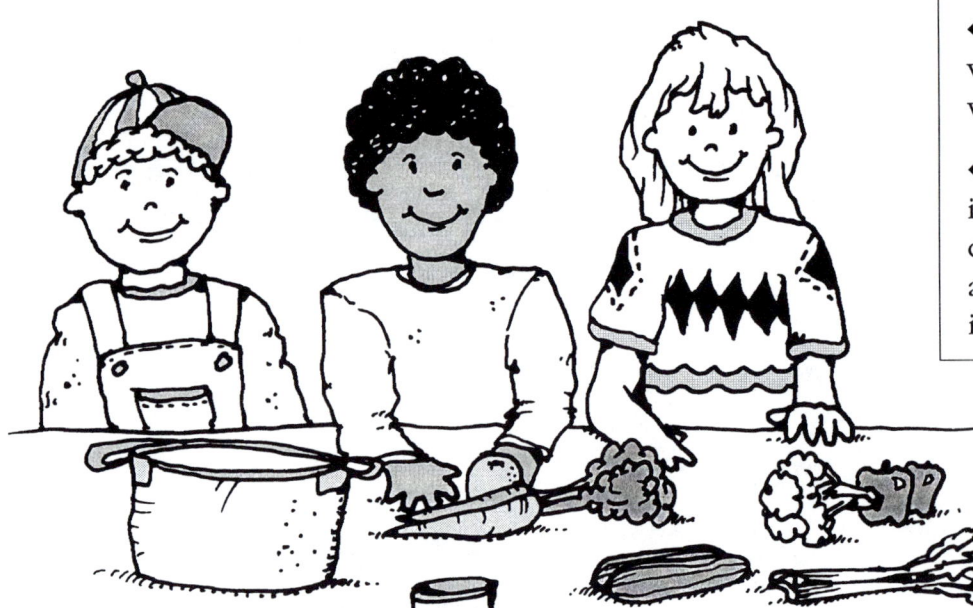

Developing Cooperation Skills

◆ Ask each child to bring a vegetable for the soup. Help your children prepare their vegetables.

◆ Set out a variety of prepared vegetables. Let your children work together to decide which vegetables to put in the soup.

◆ Ask your children to think about what the soup would taste like without any vegetables. Then ask them to think about what it would taste like if they all brought the same vegetables. Talk about how much fun it is to work together with their different likes and tastes to make something.

Buttermilk Biscuits

1 cup all-purpose flour
1 cup whole-wheat flour
2 ½ teaspoons baking powder
½ teaspoon baking soda
¼ teaspoon salt
1 tablespoon sugar
⅓ cup firm butter or margarine
¾ cup buttermilk

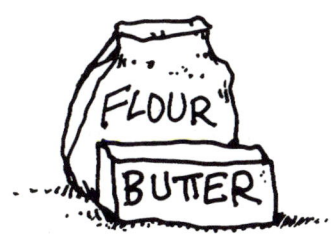

Mix the flours, baking powder, baking soda, salt, and sugar together in a bowl. Cut butter into small pieces and add them to the bowl. Use your fingers to mix butter into the dry ingredients, until the mixture is crumbly. Stir in buttermilk. Turn the dough onto a floured surface and knead 10 times. Flatten the dough into a 9-inch circle with your hands or a rolling pin. Use a biscuit cutter or an inverted glass to cut circles out of the dough. Place the circles on a greased baking sheet. Bake at 400°F for 15 to 20 minutes. Makes about twelve 2-inch biscuits.

Hint: If desired, use some of the butter and buttermilk from making Butter (recipe on page 28).

(recipe on page 28)

Cooking Skills

◆ Let your children help measure the ingredients. (For mixing them together, see activity suggestion below.)

◆ Instead of a biscuit cutter, let your children use cookie cutters to cut different shapes out of the dough.

◆ Let your children place the warm biscuits in a towel-lined basket and pass them out.

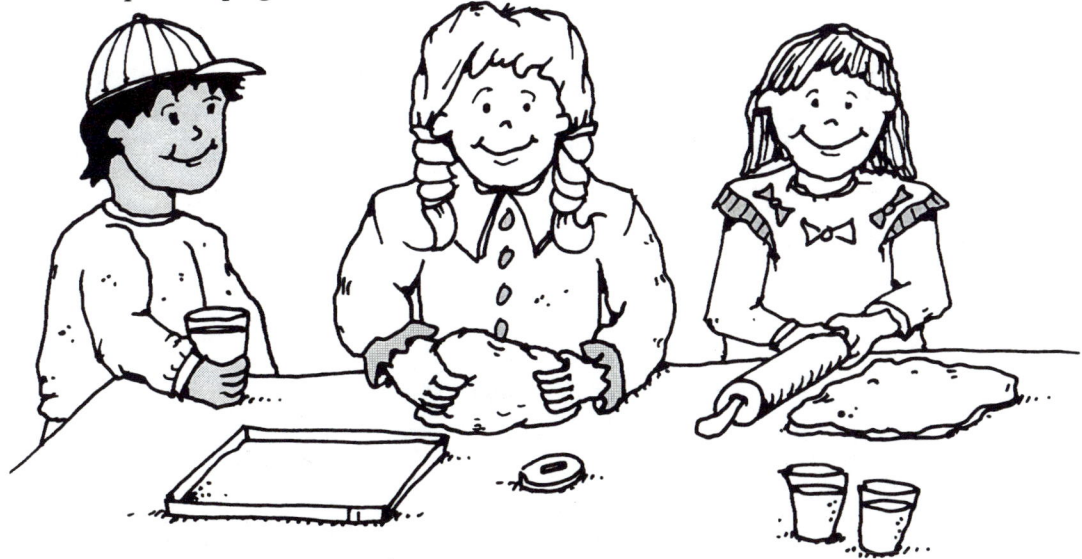

Developing Cooperation Skills

◆ Give each of your children a part of the dry ingredients. Let them put their ingredients into the bowl.

◆ Have your children take turns using their hands to mix the butter into the dry ingredients.

◆ Let your children work together to knead the dough and flatten it into a circle. Then have your children take turns using the biscuit cutter to cut out circles.

Queen-of-Hearts Tarts

Tarts:
- 1 cup all-purpose flour
- ½ teaspoon salt
- ⅔ cup shortening
- 2 to 3 tablespoons cold water

Filling:
- ⅔ cup cranberry-strawberry juice, divided
- ½ envelope (1 teaspoon) unflavored gelatin
- 1 cup vanilla yogurt

To make tarts, mix flour and salt together in a bowl. Cut in shortening with a pastry blender or your fingers. Add 2 tablespoons cold water and blend with a fork until dough forms a ball. Stir in additional water as needed. Roll out dough on a floured surface to a ⅛-inch thickness. Set out 12 muffin-tin cups. Find a drinking glass with an opening slightly larger than one of the muffin-tin cups. Use the glass to cut 12 circles out of the dough. Gently press each circle into one of the cups. Bake at 475°F for 7 to 9 minutes. Allow the tarts to cool.

To make the filling, put ⅓ cup juice in a bowl and sprinkle unflavored gelatin on top. Heat the remaining ⅓ cup juice to a boil. Pour the boiling juice on the gelatin mixture and stir until the gelatin is dissolved. Allow the mixture to cool slightly. Stir in yogurt. Pour the mixture into the cooled tarts and refrigerate for at least 2 hours. Makes 12 tarts.

Cooking Skills

◆ Let your children help measure and mix together the ingredients for the tarts and the filling.

◆ Have your children help roll and cut out the dough.

◆ Ask your children to predict what will happen to the gelatin mixture once it has been in the refrigerator.

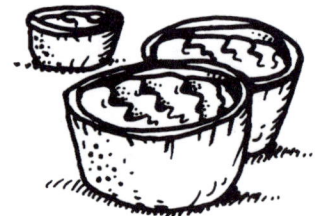

Extending Storytime

◆ Recite the rhyme "Queen of Hearts" to your children before serving these tarts.

The Queen of Hearts, she made some tarts,
All on a summer's day.
The Knave of Hearts, he stole the tarts,
And with them ran away.

The King of Hearts called for the tarts,
And scolded the Knave full score.
The Knave of Hearts brought back the tarts,
And vowed he'd steal no more.

Adapted Traditional

◆ Place the prepared tarts on a platter and hide them somewhere in your room. Explain to your children that the Knave of Hearts has just stolen the tarts and they must find them.

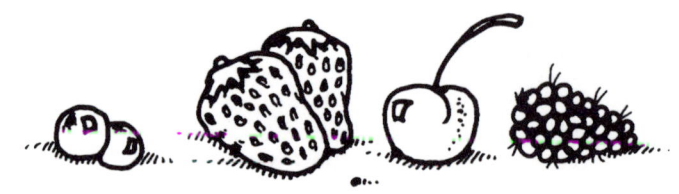

Muffin-Man Muffins

¾ cup all-purpose flour
¾ cup whole-wheat flour
1 ½ teaspoons baking powder
½ teaspoon salt
½ teaspoon cinnamon
2 tablespoons powdered milk
3 tablespoons vegetable oil
3 tablespoons pure maple syrup
1 egg
¾ cup water
½ cup raisins, chopped

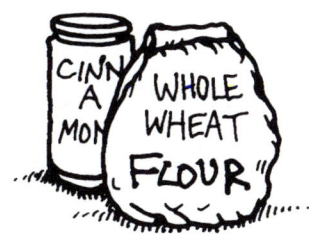

In a large bowl, stir together flours, baking powder, salt, cinnamon, and powdered milk. In a separate bowl, beat together oil, maple syrup, egg, and water. Add the wet ingredients to the dry and mix just until blended. Fold in raisins. Place paper baking cups in 12 muffin-tin cups. Fill each baking cup ⅔ full with batter. Bake at 375°F for 12 to 14 minutes. Makes 12 muffins.

Hint: Substitute 1½ cups whole-wheat pastry flour (available at health-food stores) for the all-purpose and whole-wheat flours to make a lighter-tasting muffin.

Cooking Skills

◆ Let your children help measure and mix together the ingredients.

◆ Have your children put paper baking cups in the muffin-tin cups. Help your children spoon the batter into the muffin cups.

◆ Let your children arrange the muffins on a serving tray.

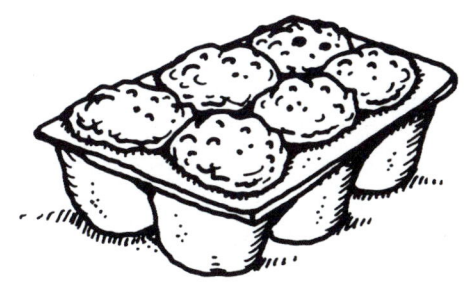

Extending Storytime

◆ Sing "The Muffin Man" with your children before eating these muffins.

Oh, do you know the muffin man,
The muffin man, the muffin man?
Oh, do you know the muffin man
Who lives in Drury Lane?

Oh, yes, I know the muffin man,
The muffin man, the muffin man.
Oh, yes, I know the muffin man
Who lives in Drury Lane.

Traditional

◆ Arrange the muffins on a tray. Ask one of your children to pretend to be the Muffin Man and pass out muffins to the other children.

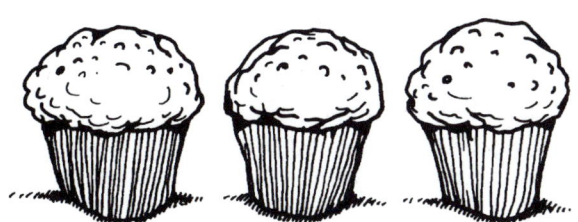

Gingerbread Kids

½ cup vegetable oil
½ cup pure maple syrup
½ cup dark molasses
1½ cups all-purpose flour
1 cup whole-wheat flour
¾ teaspoon salt
½ teaspoon soda
¾ teaspoon ginger
¼ teaspoon nutmeg
⅛ teaspoon allspice

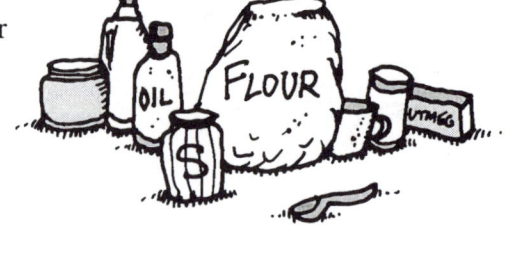

In a mixing bowl, combine oil, maple syrup, and molasses. Add the remaining ingredients and mix well. Chill the dough for 2 to 3 hours. Divide the dough in half. Roll out one half on a floured surface to a ¼-inch thickness. Cut out Gingerbread-Kid shapes. Repeat with the remaining dough. Place the shapes on baking sheets and bake at 375°F for 8 to 10 minutes. Makes 3 to 4 dozen cookies.

Cooking Skills

◆ Let your children help measure and mix together the ingredients.

◆ Give each child a small amount of dough to roll out. Let your children use Gingerbread-Kid cookie cutters to cut shapes out of their dough.

◆ When the cookies have baked, let your children use a spatula to remove them from the baking sheet.

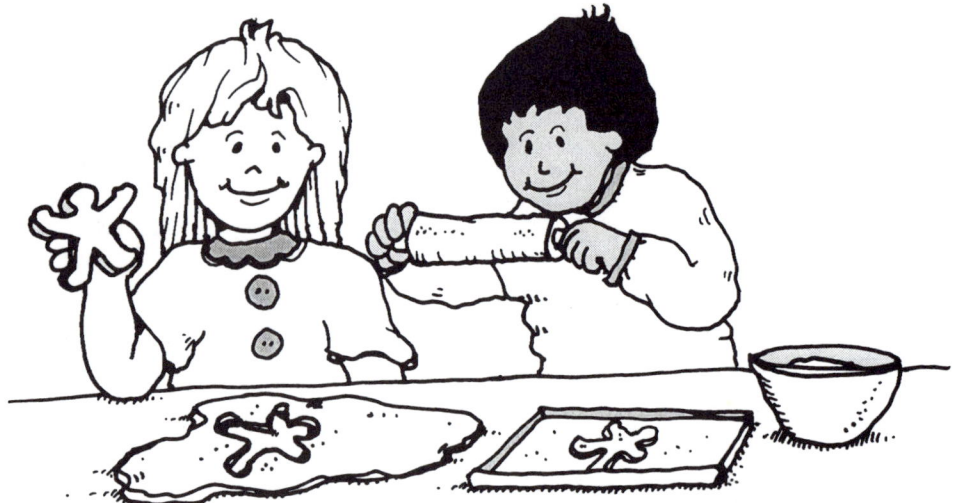

Extending Storytime

◆ Let your children help you bake the cookies. When the cookies are done baking, have someone else remove them from the oven. Secretly place a note on the outside of the oven door directing the children to another place to look for the cookies. Have another note waiting for your children in that place. Continue with as many places as desired until the children find the cookies.

◆ Read or tell your children the story of "The Gingerbread Boy" before eating the cookies.

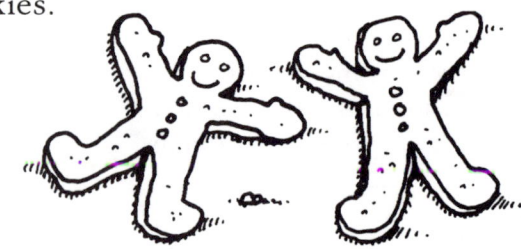

Pease Porridge

1 ½ cups dry split peas (green, yellow, or a combination
     of both)
 6 cups water
 1 bay leaf
1 ¼ teaspoons salt
 ¾ teaspoon dry mustard
 1 onion, minced
 2 stalks celery, chopped
 1 carrot, diced
 1 potato, diced

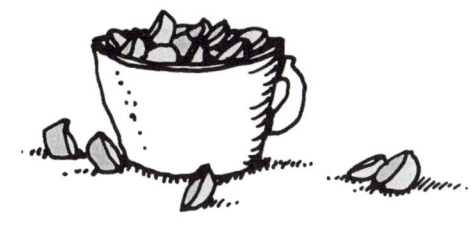

Place split peas, water, bay leaf, salt, and dry mustard in a large pan. Bring to a boil. Turn down heat and simmer for 20 minutes. Add remaining ingredients and cook for 45 minutes or until peas are soft. Remove bay leaf. Cool slightly before serving. Makes 5 ½ cups.

Cooking Skills

◆ Let your children help measure the split peas and water.

◆ Have your children help wash and prepare the vegetables for the porridge.

◆ Put the soup into a tureen. Let your children take turns using a ladle to spoon the soup into bowls.

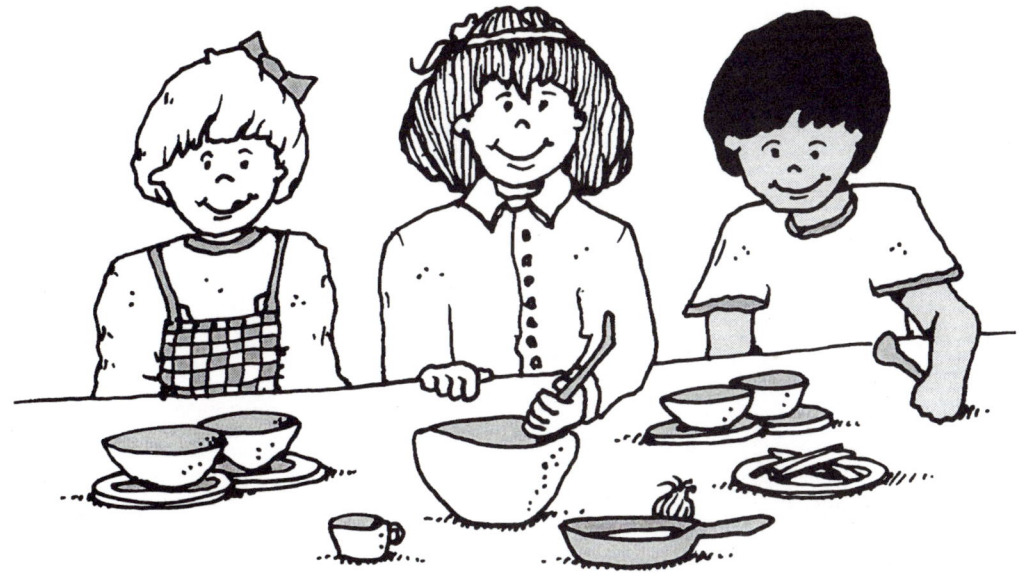

Extending Storytime

◆ Recite the rhyme "Pease Porridge Hot" with your children before eating the porridge.

Pease porridge hot, pease porridge cold,
Pease porridge in the pot, nine days old.

Some like it hot, some like it cold,
Some like it in the pot, nine days old.

Traditional

◆ Give each child a small amount of warm soup and a small amount of soup that has been chilled. Have the children taste both and decide which they like best, pease porridge hot or pease porridge cold.

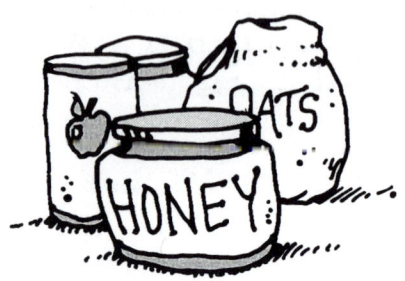

Index

TOTLINE® BOOKS

Hands-on, creative teaching ideas for parents and teachers

Activity Books

BEAR HUGS® SERIES
Remembering the Rules
Staying in Line
Circle Time
Transition Times
Time Out
Saying Goodbye

BUSY BEES SERIES
Busy Bees–Fall

PIGGYBACK® SONGS SERIES
Piggyback Songs
More Piggyback Songs
Piggyback Songs for
  Infants and Toddlers
Piggyback Songs in
  Praise of God
Piggyback Songs in
  Praise of Jesus
Holiday Piggyback Songs
Animal Piggyback Songs
Piggyback Songs
  for School
Piggyback Songs to Sign

1•2•3 SERIES
1•2•3 Art
1•2•3 Games
1•2•3 Colors
1•2•3 Puppets
1•2•3 Murals
1•2•3 Books
1•2•3 Reading & Writing
1•2•3 Rhymes, Stories
  & Songs
1•2•3 Math
1•2•3 Science

MIX & MATCH PATTERNS
Animal Patterns
Everyday Patterns
Holiday Patterns
Nature Patterns

CUT & TELL SERIES
Scissor Stories for Fall
Scissor Stories for Winter
Scissor Stories for Spring

TEACHING TALE SERIES
Teeny-Tiny Folktales
Short-Short Stories
Mini-Mini Musicals

TAKE-HOME SERIES
Alphabet & Number
  Rhymes
Color, Shape & Season
  Rhymes
Object Rhymes
Animal Rhymes

THEME-A-SAURUS® SERIES
Theme-A-Saurus
Theme-A-Saurus II
Toddler Theme-A-Saurus
Alphabet Theme-A-Saurus
Nursery Rhyme
  Theme-A-Saurus
Storytime
  Theme-A-Saurus

EXPLORING SERIES
Exploring Sand
Exploring Water
Exploring Wood

CELEBRATION SERIES
Small World Celebrations
Special Day Celebrations
Yankee Doodle
  Birthday Celebrations
Great Big Holiday
  Celebrations

LEARNING & CARING ABOUT
Our World
Our Selves
Our Town

1001 SERIES
1001 Teaching Props
1001 Teaching Tips
1001 Rhymes

ABC SERIES
ABC Space
ABC Farm
ABC Zoo
ABC Circus

PLAY & LEARN SERIES
Play & Learn
  with Magnets
Play & Learn with
  Rubber Stamps

SNACK SERIES
Super Snacks
Healthy Snacks
Teaching Snacks

More books in this series!

OTHER
Celebrating Childhood
Home Activity Booklet
23 Hands-On Workshops
Cooperation Booklet

Cut & Tell Cutouts

NURSERY TALES
The Gingerbread Kid
Henny Penny
The Three Bears
The Three Billy Goats Gruff
Little Red Riding Hood
The Three Little Pigs

NUMBER RHYMES
Hickory, Dickory Dock
Humpty Dumpty
1, 2, Buckle My Shoe
Old Mother Hubbard
Rabbit, Rabbit,
  Carrot Eater
Twinkle, Twinkle
  Little Star

Children's Books

HUFF AND PUFF SERIES
Huff and Puff's
  April Showers
Huff and Puff Around
  the World
Huff and Puff Go to School
Huff and Puff
  on Halloween
Huff and Puff
  on Thanksgiving
Huff and Puff's
  Foggy Christmas

NATURE SERIES
The Bear and
  the Mountain
Ellie the Evergreen
The Wishing Fish

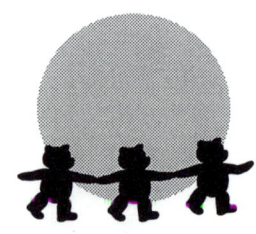

Warren Publishing House, Inc.